Preface to the

The text has been completely revised for this edition of *Pain Relief in Labour* and scarcely a page has escaped the process of up-dating. Among the numerous additions are sections on the placental transfer of drugs and references to newer drugs such as naloxone and metoclopramide. The account of epidural analgesia has been expanded because of the continued growth of the use of this technique and the closer involvement of midwives in the management of labour under epidural analgesia and in the conduct of established epidural blockade. The sections on defibrination and amniotic fluid embolism have been rewritten in the light of modern views on these topics.

There have been changes in style and format in this edition. Foetus has become fetus, not in deference to American spelling idiosyncrasy but to the Latin origin of the word. Extradural has become epidural because this has become the widely accepted term in the United Kingdom although etymological purists may prefer extradural. The lay-out of the book has been somewhat modified and is I think more pleasing. The now official, if not always welcomed, SI (Système International) units have been introduced on the assumption that their use will spread.

There is a growing awareness that narcotic analgesics and general anaesthetics will always cause a measurable degree of neonatal depression and new methods of neuro-behavioural assessment of the newborn indicate that depression of reflex activity persists for many hours after delivery. The inadequacy of narcotic analgesics for the relief of pain in many labours is being more widely acknowledged and as a corollary the use of the much more effective technique of epidural analgesia is increasing. Efforts are being made to improve the efficiency of narcotic analgesics by controlled intermittent or continuous intravenous administration.

A black spot persists in the maternal mortality rate due to general anaesthesia. From the most up to date information available over 10 per cent of the mothers who died in childbirth in England and Wales in 1970/72 died from general anaesthesia. The pulmonary aspiration of gastric contents and the resultant Mendelson's syndrome is the principal cause of these deaths. Mendelson's syndrome should be viewed as an avoidable cause of death and it is to be greatly regretted that there are even today maternity units where antacids are not routinely administered to women in labour. General anaesthesia is now one of the major causes of maternal death and regional analgesia should be substituted whenever possible.

Glasgow, 1978   Donald D. Moir

Preface to the First Edition

It is 15 years since a book devoted to the relief of pain in labour was written for midwives and published in Great Britain. Many changes have occurred in midwifery, obstetric and anaesthetic practice since 1955. Pre-mixed gases and Penthrane have been introduced and 'gas and air' analgesia has been abandoned.

The principal aim of this book is to provide the midwife with the understanding as well as the factual knowledge necessary for the best use of the various forms of analgesia available to her. As Walter Channing, the first American to use anaesthesia in childbirth said of his own Treatize on Etherization in Childbirth 'it treats of a noble subject – the remedy of pain'. The midwife has at her disposal a number of methods of analgesia which, if used to advantage, are capable of giving a substantial measure of pain relief in normal labour.

I have tried to adopt a scientific, rather than an emotional approach to subjects which are capable of arousing strong emotional responses. I have emphasised important principles and have tried to avoid dogmatic statements where these are not justified by the available evidence. Where doubt exists I have offered what I believe to be the correct answer, although time may prove me wrong.

I have described and explained a number of procedures which are not normally carried out by midwives, but which are in use in maternity hospitals. I believe that a midwife should understand the procedures which she sees performed on her patients. Only in this way can she give the highest standards of patient care and maintain her interest in her chosen profession. I have devoted a chapter to local anaesthesia and regional analgesia, because midwives may now use local anaesthetics for perineal infiltration and because techniques such as extradural analgesia and paracervical block are now used in many hospitals and their use is likely to increase. The care of the patient in labour and the detection of the complications of regional analgesia remain a responsibility of the midwife.

I have included considerable detail on the subjects of resuscitation and general anaesthesia. General anaesthesia is widely used for operative delivery in British hospitals and is now a major cause of maternal death. The midwife has an important contribution to make towards reducing the disturbingly high death rate due to general anaesthesia by enforcing a proper dietary regime and administering alkalis to her patients during labour. An operative delivery rate of 30 per cent or higher is common in British hospitals and often about half of these operations take place under general anaesthesia.

The midwife, the obstetrician and the anaesthetist can all contribute to the relief of pain in labour. There is no room for interprofessional rivalries and prejudices. As Sir James Young Simpson wrote in 1848, 'It is our duty as well as our privilege to use all legitimate means to mitigate and remove the physical sufferings of the mother during parturition'. The midwife will usually be in the best position to relieve the pain of normal labour. She has the advantage of close personal contact with her patient and has a number of new, safe and quite effective drugs and techniques at her command.

I am sincerely grateful to all the midwives, obstetricians, anaesthetists and patients from whom I have learned something about the relief of pain in labour and I am especially appreciative of the enlightened attitude of the obstetricians and midwives in the Queen Mother's Hospital, Glasgow towards the introduction of newer methods, such as continuous extradural analgesia.

My thanks are due to Mrs Jeanette MacInnes for typing the manuscript, to Mr Gabriel Donald of the Western Infirmary, Glasgow for the illustrations and to Miss Dorothy Officer, Senior Tutor and Dr James Willocks, Consultant Obstetrician at the Queen Mother's Hospital for helpful criticism of the text.

My adviser and my constant helper has been my wife, who is herself a midwife and a mother and to her I am especially grateful for her knowledge, experience and encouragement.

Glasgow, 1971   Donald D. Moir

Contents

Contents

1 History

The outstanding event in the history of pain relief in childbirth was the first administration of ether for a delivery by Doctor (later Sir) James Young Simpson in Edinburgh in January, 1847. The operation was internal podalic version and the delivery of a dead fetus from a patient with severe pelvic contracture. Simpson, then 36 years old, was the son of a village baker and had become holder of the oldest European chair of midwifery at the age of 29.

Ether had been used in Boston in October, 1846 by William T. G. Morton and anaesthesia was soon to be known as the Yankee Dodge. Even earlier, in 1844, Horace Wells of Hartford, Connecticut had used nitrous oxide in dentistry but unfortunately his public demonstration in Boston was a failure and Wells was hissed from the room by the medical students. It was many years before the use of nitrous oxide was revived.

Simpson, however, gets the credit for the first obstetric anaesthetic. Simpson was dissatisfied with the slow induction associated with open ether anaesthesia and tried numerous other chemicals on himself, his assistants and his family, often seated at the dinner table. In November, 1847 he discovered the anaesthetic properties of chloroform when his assistants, Matthews Duncan and George Keith, fell to the floor after inhaling this substance. Simpson soon administered the first chloroform anaesthetics to his patients.

For the next 100 years ether and chloroform remained the principal, indeed almost the sole, anaesthetic agents in use in midwifery. Chloroform was dropped on to an open mask or a handkerchief and when used as an analgesic a few drops were administered with each uterine contraction. This type of analgesia was administered to Queen Victoria in 1853 much to the satisfaction of that experienced multipara and this method of intermittent inhalational analgesia became known as chloroform à la reine. The early years of anaesthesia saw powerful opposition to the idea of relieving pain in labour by many clergymen and not a few doctors. This opposition was based on the text from Genesis: 'In sorrow thou shalt bring forth children'. Simpson's pen and tongue and royal patronage finally overcame this opposition.

Until 1847 there had been no really effective methods of anaesthesia or analgesia. From Ancient Egyptian and Babylonian times attempts had been made to relieve the pains of labour and delivery but these efforts can have met with little success. Any success probably depended more on faith than on pharmacological efficacy and most methods could be broadly classified as psychological, perhaps involving an element of hypnotism in some instances. Other methods, still in use by a few primitive tribes, were definitely physical, such as those which involved jumping on the maternal abdomen to hasten delivery and relieve pain.

From earliest times pain was often regarded as being due to the presence of evil spirits or demons which might be dispelled by charms and incantations. Christianity brought with it a concept of pain as a divine punishment and a means of achieving Grace through suffering. Attempts at pain relief were sometimes condemned by religious authorities as being contrary to the will of God, an attitude still present in Simpson's time. Witchcraft was sometimes invoked for the banishment of demons from the patient's body. In 1591 Eufame MacCalzean was burned alive in Edinburgh, without the mercy of previous strangling, having been found guilty of 28 charges of witchcraft. One charge was the use of charms to cast the pains of labour on to a dog which ran away and was never seen again.

The conditions under which midwifery was practised before 1847 are difficult for us, who are accustomed to regard surgery and anaesthesia as inseparable, to imagine. Labour often lasted for many days to be terminated by a destructive operation or the death of the mother and the suffering must have been dreadful indeed. In 1848 the humanitarian Simpson said 'The distress and pain which women often endure while they are struggling through a difficult labour are beyond description and seem to be more than human nature would be able to bear under any other circumstance'.

Since Simpson's great discovery many new agents and techniques have been introduced. Chloroform and ether have now been almost replaced by anaesthetics which are less likely to cause respiratory depression in the newborn and are less likely to cause atonic postpartum haemorrhage. The newer methods are usually more pleasant for the mother and, in skilled hands, are safer. Where facilities or money are limited the older methods are simple and inexpensive and are safer for anaesthetists experienced in their use and inexperienced with more complex techniques. Chloroform is capable of causing sudden death from ventricular fibrillation.

The early history of anaesthesia is international and later developments too came from many countries. Among the important milestones were the first use of nitrous oxide in midwifery by the Russian Klikowitch in 1880. Spinal (subarachnoid) analgesia was introduced by Bier of Germany in 1898 and, although now seldom used in British obstetrics, spinal analgesia is extensively used in other parts of the world, including North America, for forceps delivery and Caesarean section. In France, in 1901, Sicard and Cathélin, each working independently in Paris, introduced single injection caudal epidural analgesia. The development of continuous caudal and lumbar epidural analgesia by indwelling epidural catheter, by Hingson and Edwards in the U.S.A. in 1942, laid the foundations for the current widespread use of caudal and lumbar epidural analgesia in North America and for the recent welcome interest in these most effective methods of analgesia in the United Kingdom. Regional analgesia has deservedly become popular in recent years and pudendal block and epidural block are now the commonest forms of anaesthesia for forceps delivery. Paracervical block, popularised over the last 10 years in the U.S.A. and to a lesser extent in the United Kingdom, is now rarely used because of the occurrence of fetal bradycardia and intrauterine death in association with this otherwise simple and valuable method of first stage analgesia. Recently midwives have been permitted to infiltrate the perineum with local anaesthetic before episiotomy.

Many systemic analgesics are, or have been, used in

midwifery. Outstanding events were the isolation of morphine from crude opium by Serturner in 1806 and, of great practical significance, the invention of the hypodermic syringe and hollow needle by Alexander Wood of Edinburgh in 1853. Until then the injection of drugs had been difficult and rarely undertaken. Morphine and hyoscine (Scopolamine) were used in Germany in 1902 to produce twilight sleep. This involved analgesia and sedation together with amnesia, so that patients were unable to recall the events of labour. Twilight sleep is seldom used today because it causes respiratory depression in the newborn and tends to cause delirium and restlessness in the mother. Pethidine was synthesised in 1939 and approved for midwives' use in 1950, thus placing for the first time a potent analgesic drug in the hands of midwives. Pentazocine was approved for use by midwives in 1972.

Inhalational methods are of course extensively used by midwives for analgesia in labour. In 1933 R. J. Minnitt, a Liverpool anaesthetist, designed his apparatus for the administration of nitrous oxide and air. In 1936 the Midwives Boards approved the use of this apparatus by midwives. Despite the fact that 'gas and air' analgesia must inevitably produce some degree of maternal and fetal hypoxia, the Minnitt's and kindred apparatus have given pain relief to millions of women with apparent safety in most instances. Withdrawal of recognition of this apparatus in April, 1970, marks the end of an era of hypoxic analgesia. (The Central Midwives Board for Scotland withdrew its approval in December, 1969). Nitrous oxide is now always given with oxygen and analgesia is administered by the Entonox apparatus, developed by Tunstall of Aberdeen and others and given C. M. B. approval in 1965, and by the Lucy Baldwin apparatus. Trilene, although introduced as an anaesthetic in 1941, was not approved for use by midwives until 1955. Methoxyflurane (Penthrane), a relatively new agent with properties akin to Trilene, was approved in 1970 by the C. M. B. for England and may be marginally superior to Trilene. The use of methoxyflurane was approved by the C. M. B. for Scotland in 1972.

The value of psychological preparation for labour has been stressed by Grantly Dick Read since 1933 when he postulated the Fear-Tension-Pain syndrome. Although Read's claims have not been fully substantiated by others, the value of antenatal preparation for childbirth is generally recognised. Among the many schemes of preparation the psychoprophylaxis method based on the work of Lamaze and Vellay of France over the past 20 years is now accepted by many as being of value.

Present methods of general anaesthesia for obsetrics are based on the work of the late Hamer Hodges of Portsmouth who, in 1959, demonstrated the superiority of light thiopentone, nitrous oxide and muscle relaxant anaesthesia over older methods. This type of anaesthesia has minimal effects on the fetus, is more pleasant for the mother and is safe in skilled hands. In Great Britain obstetric anaesthesia is nearly always administered by a specialist anaesthetist. Unfortunately these high risk anaesthetics are too often delegated to junior anaesthetists. It is distressing to record that the maternal mortality due to general anaesthesia has recently risen in Great Britain. Currently about 10 per cent of maternal deaths are due directly to anaesthesia. There is need for the expansion of obstetric anaesthetic services and the more frequent provision of a 24 hour resident anaesthetic service for major maternity units. With such a service would come an increased use of techniques such as continuous epidural analgesia in labour and consequently really effective pain relief would then be available to those patients whose pain is inadequately relieved by simpler methods.

2. Psychoprophylaxis and Allied Methods

In this chapter it is proposed to consider the various methods of antenatal preparation for childbirth which are based on the inculcation of a proper attitude to labour and often also involve a series of exercises designed to encourage relaxation during contractions and sometimes to strengthen muscles used at delivery. The belief that childbearing is a pleasurable experience is promoted. Hypnosis and methods such as the use of White Sound and the Heyns' decompression suit which are based, at least in part, on distraction therapy are also included.

Space does not permit a detailed description of these methods, nor does the author feel competent to undertake this task. A short list of suggested further reading for those specially interested in these techniques is given at the end of this chapter.

It is difficult for anyone, either patient or professional attendant, to take an unbiased view of these methods. Many factors colour the attitudes of all of us and these factors are almost impossible to eliminate in any attempt at scientific assessment of a method of psychological preparation for labour. Opinions vary from the wildly enthusiastic to the frankly derisory. The influence of an enthusiastic teacher may be paramount and long ingrained social and racial influences must affect individual responses. There is also the well recognised placebo response whereby, in the field of analgesic drug therapy, a completely inert tablet or injection can be expected to relieve pain in about 30 per cent of patients who expect pain relief. Thus the very anticipation that a form of 'treatment' will produce a certain effect means that this effect will often by produced. Yet, if there is no prior psychological preparation there is no effect. This statement does not of course detract from the value of the therapy for the patient. It is therefore important for the patient that midwives and doctors, even if not themselves enthusiasts for a method, should do nothing to destroy the patient's faith in her chosen regime. The attendants should also have a general knowledge of the various methods which may be used by their patients. The mode of action of these methods is uncertain but faith, understanding and perhaps distraction by the performance of various exercises may all play a part in altering the patient's response to the stimulus of a uterine contraction. Distraction may also be a factor in inhalational analgesia while profound relaxation may produce a state apparently akin to hypnosis.

It is my firm belief that painless labour should never be promised to any patient who undertakes to study and practise a method of psychological preparation for labour. I believe that a considerable percentage of women can obtain a valuable reduction in the total amount of pain experienced in labour by a suitable preparation and that antenatal instruction in the process of labour is never wasted. It should be explained to the patient that, despite her best efforts, she may experience pain in labour. The fault is neither her own, nor necessarily that of the method in which she believed until then. She should not be allowed to feel that she has somehow failed and must be ready to accept other forms of analgesia should they be needed. In my opinion there is no need for the clash which sometimes undoubtedly occurs between the proponents of the psychological and pharmacological approaches to analgesia. The two approaches should be complementary and there should be no hesitation in accepting an analgesic drug or an epidural block if the results of a psychological regime are not completely satisfactory. It should be remembered that there are obstetric conditions, such as an occipito-posterior position, cephalo-pelvic disproportion or incoordinate uterine action, which may cause unusually prolonged and painful labour in which powerful methods of pain relief may be required.

Patients who receive special preparation are a self-selecting group and perhaps more likely to be intelligent, healthy and concerned for the welfare of their infants. They are predisposed to believe in the method. It may be unfair to compare results achieved in this type of patient with those experienced in a group of patients who have had no antenatal preparation.

The avoidance of, or the reduced need for, analgesic drugs in labour is likely to reduce the incidence of respiratory depression in the newborn. Another advantage of antenatal instruction is that in hospital practice the patient becomes more familiar with her new surroundings and gets to know the people who will look after her in labour.

On balance, psychological preparation for labour is never without value. The results may occasionally be dramatic, the knowledge of the process of labour is never wasted and almost every woman can obtain some significant help, but, despite the enthusiasm of some teachers, the individual patient should not expect certain, painless labour.

Techniques of Psychological Preparation for Labour

Almost every maternity unit has its own methods of preparing patients for labour and often borrows details and concepts from more than one recognised scheme. There is no harm in this if the teacher can communicate her knowledge and enthusiasm to her patients. Usually a course of about six or eight classes is offered to patients attending the antenatal clinic. In all such courses instruction in the elementary physiology of labour and in mothercraft should be included. A simple account of systemic, inhalational and, where appropriate, epidural analgesia should be offered and inhalational analgesia apparatus should be demonstrated. Epidural analgesia should not be regarded as a technique solely for use in abnormal labours but should be presented as a particularly effective method of pain relief. The patient is of course at liberty to reject this, or any other technique of analgesia. In addition, a series of exercises is usually taught. According to the policy of the clinic, these exercises may be designed principally to teach the mother to relax during labour and commonly include breathing exercises to be performed in the first and second stages. Additionally in some schemes there are exercises designed to improve posture, relieve backache and to strengthen muscles used at delivery. Diet and hygiene in pregnancy are discussed. The possibility of instrumental delivery in the best interests of mother and child is mentioned.

There are two leading methods of antenatal preparation in current use and although the protagonists of each may regard their chosen method as quite distinct from the other, it seems to the uncommitted observer that the methods have much in common and that borrowing and interchange of ideas are permissible.

The husband should be encouraged to be with his wife during labour and he too will usually benefit from simple antenatal explanation and preparation. Many hospitals now hold classes for fathers-to-be. In the past many women have felt alone in labour in strange surroundings and would have welcomed the husband's presence. The husband is likely to be distressed if his wife does not receive adequate pain relief and epidural analgesia is usually very satisfactory in this situation.

Natural childbirth

The Grantly Dick Read or Natural Childbirth method dates from 1935 and is based on the idea that fear, tension and pain are linked together. Fear is the result of ignorance of the events and processes of childbirth. Fear in turn produces tension in the muscles, including presumably the muscles of the lower pole of the uterus. This tension results in pain and in delay in labour. This vicious circle of fear-tension-pain can be broken by giving simple explanations of the birth process during pregnancy. Read taught that childbirth should be a joy. Read's theory, which is by no means generally accepted, was evolved from observing that many (but not all) women of primitive tribes seemed to suffer little or no pain in labour. He called this natural childbirth, and believed that the women had not acquired an unnatural fear of labour, unlike their civilised sisters. The Read method fell into disrepute in some circles because too much was claimed for it. The physiotherapist Helen Heardman became an enthusiastic advocate of natural childbirth and taught women to prepare mentally and physically for labour as an athlete trains for a race. Women were encouraged to strive for painless labour and spontaneous delivery and if either of these objectives was not attained then a profound sense of failure sometimes followed. Only the exceptional patient has a painless labour and the reactions of a patient who has believed in the method and then experiences pain may be violent, disturbing and disappointing. Commonly this philosophy is accompanied by a series of relaxation exercises which are practised antenatally and in labour. At 'relaxation classes' a peaceful atmosphere is provided in a semi-darkened room and the mothers are taught to relax all their muscles while in the dorsal and semi-prone positions. The teacher speaks quietly, suggests pleasant thoughts and relaxation by her every word. It is interesting to note that the technique of hypnosis is very similar and indeed it is quite common for patients to fall asleep at the classes.

Psychoprophylaxis

The method of psychoprophylaxis was developed in France by Lamaze in 1956 and Vellay in 1960 and was based on earlier Russian work. An underlying concept is that of the conditioned reflex as demonstrated by Pavlov. It is held that most women have been conditioned to believe that uterine contractions are painful. The first task is therefore deconditioning until this belief is no longer held and this is followed by reconditioning to the idea that contractions need not be painful. It may be pointed out to the woman that contracting a skeletal muscle is not painful and she may be shown how to feel her own painless Braxton Hicks contractions.

Emphasis is placed on active patient participation. Instruction in the physiology of labour is provided and the fact that labour may be abnormal is accepted. A series of exercises is practised. Many of these are breathing exercises and types A, B, C and D breathing are taught for use during contractions of increasing intensity. A potential danger of extreme overbreathing is that it may lower the maternal blood carbon dioxide tension to levels which may reduce placental blood flow and cause fetal hypoxia and acidosis. Although hyperventilation to such an extent is not advocated, nevertheless it may happen and the midwife should discourage sustained overbreathing. Maternal tetany, taking the form of muscular twitching, may be precipitated by overbreathing.

Painless labour is claimed for about 35 per cent of patients who practice psychoprophylaxis. It is also claimed that for the 65 per cent who have pain, the pain may be lessened and that self-control is unlikely to be lost. This is important for most women (and their attendants). Psychoprophylaxis seems to me to offer a more realistic approach than the older Read method. Most women find it of definite value and the acceptance that labour may be abnormal and sometimes painful enough to require the use of other forms of analgesia is sound.

Hypnosis

Hypnosis, too, has its advantages. Although the mechanisms of hypnotism are uncertain there is nothing very mysterious about the technique which is quite simple. The patient lies down in quiet and comforable surroundings and the hypnotist suggests relaxation and sleep. A state of increased suggestibility is induced and the patient is then told that labour will be painless or at least less painful. Gadgets and gimmicks are not employed. Only adults of reasonable intelligence who are willing subjects are suitable for this approach to the ideal of painless labour. About 25 per cent of patients can be hypnotised to a level at which the appreciation of pain is abolished or substantially reduced. The comparison between the technique of hypnotism and some of the methods used in 'relaxtion classes' has already been made. In midwifery practice a hypnosis clinic may be organised and patients are then usually taught self-hypnosis, so that the present of the hypnotist is not required during labour. The success rate of hypnosis is not too different from that claimed for psychoprophylaxis (14 per cent and 59 per cent had pain-free labours in two series). A major problem is that of organising a clinic and familiarising doctors and midwives with the management of hypnotised patients. Personal choice on the patient's part is relevant and faith in this method is just as necessary as it is for psychoprophylaxis or natural childbirth. Very occasionally hypnosis may produce disastrous effects in a patient who is already psychiatrically disturbed and the possibility of after effects on normal patients has not been absolutely excluded.

Abdominal decompression

In 1955 Heyns of South Africa introduced the technique of abdominal decompression as a method of reducing, although not necessarily abolishing pain in labour. The patient's lower chest, abdomen and thighs are enclosed in a plastic shell or bag (the Heyns' bag) which is sealed at its upper and lower ends. A powerful suction is applied with each contraction so that a substantial negative pressure is created within the shell or bag. An electric motor is used and the patient herself controls the suction action by placing her finger over a hole in the air pipe. Heyns believes that abdominal decompression relaxes the anterior abdominal wall. It is said that the upper segment of the uterus becomes more spherical and acts in a more efficient manner. Labour is shortened and less painful. It has been claimed that 85 per cent of patients in one series obtained good or excellent relief of pain.

Abdominal decompression appears to involve muscular relaxation, powerful distraction therapy, a large measure of enthusiasm on the part of its advocates and a more physiological type of uterine action. The apparatus itself is impressive to most patients. In the Queen Mother's Hospital it was found that some patients were terrified of the apparatus and of the noise of the electric motor and begged to be removed from the decompression bag. With the plastic shells there may be a feeling of constriction around the chest, diminished venous return from the legs and the suction may cause liquor amnii to drain in an unpleasant manner. Abdominal decompression must of course be discontinued in the second stage of labour. Access to the abdomen for palpation and auscultation of the fetal heart is difficult with some types of apparatus. Nevertheless, patients who find the method acceptable can achieve a substantial measure of pain relief.

Other, more sensational, claims have been made for abdominal decompression. For example, it has been suggested that its regular use in the antenatal period may improve uteroplacental blood flow, increase fetal oxygenation and even produce more intelligent babies. These claims must await objective assessment before being accepted. Valid assessment is difficult because, as with other methods of preparation for childbirth, there is a tendency for relatively intelligent women to practise the technique and one must beware of comparing the results, whether in terms of pain relief or the intelligence of offspring, with the results in a series of unprepared women.

White sound

White sound is a mixture of sounds of many frequencies. The analogy is with the colour white, which is composed of all the colours of the rainbow. White sound is sometimes likened to that of rushing water. The patient increases the volume of sound during contractions. This is probably yet another form of distraction therapy which has been used on a limited scale for pain relief in dentistry and in midwifery.

Acupuncture

Acupuncture has been used, sometimes with remarkable success in the treatment of many types of pain and in China it is sometimes used for major surgery. Acupuncture is non-toxic and would be attractive as a method of pain relief in labour, were it to prove effective. Unfortunately acupuncture failed to provide adequate analgesia to even a single member of a group of volunteer American mothers. The doctors who conducted this trial commented that acupuncture seemed not to be used in labour in China, the country of its origin.

FURTHER READING

Dick-Read, G. (1968) *Childbirth Without Fear*, 5th. edn., London: Heinemann.

Heardman, H. (1975) *Relaxation and Exercise for Natural Childbirth*, 4th. edn., Edinburgh: Churchill Livingstone.

Montgomery, E. (1969) *At Your Best for Birth and Later*, 3rd. edn., Bristol: Wright.

3. Analgesics, Sedatives and Tranquillisers — General Principles

In this chapter the general principles of the drug treatment of pain and anxiety in labour will be discussed. A sound understanding of the action of the various groups of drugs available is more important than a detailed knowledge of the pharmacology of a long list of individual drugs. When the general principles have been grasped it will then be clear that the choice of a specific drug sometimes depends more on individual preference than on any major differences between the drugs in a given group. A short list of drugs whose action is well understood is sufficient for most purposes.

The narcotic analgesics together with sedatives, tranquillisers, inhalational analgesia and some form of antenatal preparation consitute the analgesic regime for the majority of British patients. Ideally other forms of analgesia should be available for use when required, but regrettably in many British hospitals other methods are not available.

The administration of effective doses of analgesics and sedatives can never be completely safe for the mother and her infant. The most important side-effects are respiratory depression and hypotension and the benefits of pain relief have to be weighed against the potential dangers of the treatment. Some depression of reflex activity in the newborn is the usual result of the administration of analgesics and sedatives in labour.

All the powerful analgesics, with the possible exception of pentazocine (Fortral) are drugs of addiction. The risk of producing drug addiction by the administration of these drugs to a normal patient during labour is negligible, but the midwife who has access to these drugs should be aware of the addictive properties of the analgesics and to a lesser extent of the sedatives, hypnotics and tranquillisers.

Terms such as sedative, hypnotic, tranquilliser, narcotic and analgesic are used, sometimes incorrectly, and it is appropriate to define these terms at this point.

Definitions

A Sedative. This is a drug capable of relieving anxiety and inducing a feeling of calmness.

A Hypnotic. This is a drug capable of inducing sleep, resembling natural sleep. Frequently a larger dose of a sedative will act as a hypnotic.

A Tranquilliser. This is a drug capable of relieving anxiety. The distinction between a transquilliser and a sedative is not great. A tranquilliser does not usually cause drowsiness in the way that a sedative may often do.

A Narcotic. This is a drug capable of producing insensibility in sufficient dosage. The dose of a narcotic drug determines its action. A small dose of a barbiturate acts as a sedative, a larger dose acts as a hypnotic, and a yet larger dose acts as a narcotic. The term narcotic as used in pharmacology is a wide one and includes, for example, the barbiturates, the narcotic analgesics such as morphine and pethidine and also the general anaesthetics. Confusion may arise because the term narcotic is also used in a restricted sense to embrace only a defined list of drugs of addiction, e.g. morphine or pethidine.

An Analgesic. This is a drug capable of relieving pain without producing unconsciousness. The powerful analgesics such as morphine and pethidine are known as narcotic analgesics because large doses can produce insensibility. Smaller doses produce sedation or hypnosis together with analgesia. Not all narcotics are analgesics although the powerful analgesics are all narcotics. This distinction is fundamental to the correct choice of drug for a given situation. The barbiturates and chloral hydrate act as sedative or hypnotic drugs and can produce unconsciousness in large doses. They are not analgesics and should not be given to a patient who is in pain unless an analgesic drug is also prescribed. The administration of a sedative or hypnotic drug alone to a patient in pain may cause disorientation and loss of self control.

Amnesia. Amnesia means loss of memory. Certain drugs including the phenothiazine derivatives, diazepam (Valium) and hyoscine (Scopolamine) sometimes cause temporary amnesia. An interesting philosophy is sometimes propounded that the suffering of pain is of small importance, provided that the patient retains no conscious memory of her suffering. This somewhat callous concept was formerly implemented in twilight sleep. In this now obsolete regime hyoscine was administered repeatedly during labour, although only one dose of morphine was given. Patients thus managed were often in obvious pain during labour but because they did not remember this pain they would approach a subsequent labour with equanimity. Loss of memory for an unpleasant experience seems harmless and even to be desired. It is the suppression of such memories which may be harmful.

Anaesthesia. Anaesthesia implies a reversible depression of all the senses.

Therapeutic efficiency and placental transfer

Two important generalisations can be made about the drug treatment of pain and anxiety in labour.

1. There is an optimum therapeutic dose of each drug for each patient. This does lies between the dose which is too small to be of significant worth and a larger dose which, although usually more effective, is associated with too many unpleasant or dangerous side effects. Pethidine 50 mg is a safe but not very effective analgesic in labour, while pethidine 200 mg may produce good pain relief accompanied by respiratory depression, hypotension and vomiting. The optimum dose of a drug is the minimum dose capable of producing the desired effect.

2. There is no sedative, hypnotic, analgesic or anaesthetic drug which does not cross the placenta and act upon the fetus to some degree. The free placental transfer of drugs is the other great limiting factor in the management of pain in labour.

For the above two reasons efforts at pain relief in childbirth must compromise between analgesic efficiency and an element of risk for the mother and her child. The ideal analgesic for labour would be one which did not cross the placental barrier. Unfortunately no such analgesic drug exists and indeed may never be discovered. This is because analgesics, sedatives and anaesthetics act upon the mother's brain. To reach the brain they must first cross the so-called blood-brain barrier. With respect to drug transfer the properties of the blood-brain barrier are similar to those of the placental barrier so that any drug which can reach the mother's brain can also reach the fetus. Commonly the level of drugs in the fetal blood is about 70 per cent of the level in the maternal blood.

The principal properties of anaesthetics, analgesics, sedatives and tranquillisers which, without exception, permit their free placental transfer are (1) their solubility in lipids (2) their poorly ionised state in the blood (3) their lack of binding to maternal plasma proteins and (4) their low molecular weight. The concentration gradient between maternal and fetal blood is also of great importance. An intravenous injection of, for example, pethidine or thiopentone (Pentothal) produces a high concentration of drug in the mother's blood and placental transfer is rapid and extensive. Placental blood flow and placental function are also of importance.

Detoxication of drugs

Almost all narcotic drugs are broken down in the liver into inactive metabolites which are then excreted in the urine or in the faeces. In the case of volatile or gaseous agents such as Trilene or nitrous oxide excretion is mainly by the lungs.

If the liver is damaged then detoxication of drugs may be impaired and the action of drugs may be prolonged. Liver damage of this extent is rare in pregnancy. The high oestrogen levels of pregnancy can modify the breakdown of drugs in the liver and so affect the action of drugs such as pethidine, but the practical significance of this is probably small. More important is the fact that the immature liver of the fetus and newborn is not able to detoxicate drugs efficiently until several weeks after birth and the action of narcotic drugs may be very prolonged. The elimination of barbiturates may take three or four days in the newborn. Neurobehavioural testing of neonates clearly demonstrates that infants whose mothers had received pethidine have depression of reflex activity, including sucking, for up to 24 hours after birth and such infants differ quite markedly from those whose mothers received no analgesics or who received epidural analgesia.

Respiratory depression

The most important side-effect of the narcotic drugs is respiratory depression. By this we mean that these drugs are capable of acting on the respiratory centre in the brain stem of the mother and the infant so that the rate and depth of respiration are reduced. If a gross overdose of a narcotic drug is given then apnoea (complete cessation of breathing) may result.

Severe repiratory depression is uncommon in the mother, probably because the pain of uterine contractions is often accompanied by voluntary or involuntary hyperventilation. Respiratory depression may occur between contractions and cause mild hypoxia. The stimulant effect of pain is the explanation of the well-known aphorism that 'pain is the best antidote to morphine'.

The major risk is that respiratory depression in the infant at birth, caused by narcotics administered during labour to the mother, may inhibit the establishment of adequate ventilation and cause hypoxia in the newborn. Drug-induced respiratory depression in the newborn is most likely to occur when delivery takes place between one and three hours after the intramuscular administration of the drug to the mother, but is difficult to forecast with accuracy in any particular patient. Premature infants are more likely to develop respiratory depression than mature infants. It is worth repeating that in equi-analgesic doses no single narcotic analgesic is significantly less likely to produce respiratory depression than any other.

The dangers of respiratory depression due to narcotic analgesics have been lessened with the introduction of narcotic antagonists which are discussed later in this chapter. There are no effective antagonists to the barbiturates, the phenothiazines or the general anaesthetic agents.

Hypotension

The narcotic analgesics, sedatives and tranquillisers rarely cause serious hypotension after the intramuscular administration of normal doses. Rapid intravenous injection may cause a sudden precipitous fall in blood pressure. Intravenous injections should be given slowly over 5 to 10 minutes and the drug should be diluted before injection. Continuous very dilute infusions of pethidine are much safer than even slow single injections. Patients who have a reduced blood volume due to haemorrhage or excessive fluid loss from the gastro-intestinal tract are liable to develop hypotension when narcotic drugs are given.

Hypotension, if it occurs, is usually orthostatic. That is to say, the blood pressure may be adequate while the patient lies down, but if an erect or sitting posture is assumed then hypotension occurs due to pooling of blood in the dependent parts of the body. Consequently patients who have received narcotic drugs should remain in bed.

There may be an excessive fall in blood pressure if an epidural or spinal (subarachnoid) block is performed after the administration of large doses of narcotic analgesics.

Hypotension, although not without danger for the mother, may be even more dangerous for the fetus. Hypotension may reduce placental blood flow and thus impair the oxygen supply to the fetus. Maternal hypotension can cause fetal death. It is not possible to state the critical blood pressure below which the fetus is in danger because this pressure will vary from patient to patient, but most certainly the mother's blood pressure should not remain below 80 mmHg (11kPa) systolic for long.

The immediate treatment of hypotension should include turning the patient on to her left side to relieve any compression of the inferior vena cava. Raising the legs above the level of the trunk may be effective because this will give a temporary auto-transfusion of blood from the legs.

Gastro-intestinal effects

Apart from a tendency to cause constipation there are two important effects of the narcotic analgesics upon the gastro-intestinal tract.

Pethidine, morphine and allied drugs delay gastric emptying. A patient may retain food in her stomach for many hours. Should she require a general anaesthetic the risk of vomiting or regurgitation of stomach contents is high. The traditional idea that general anaesthesia may be safely administered four hours after the last meal is completely invalid where women in labour are concerned and solid food should never be given once labour is established. The aspiration of stomach contents into the lungs during general anaesthesia is now a major cause of maternal death. Metoclopramide (Maxolon) has been successfuly used to accelerate gastric emptying in labour but is probably ineffective when delay is due to narcotic analgesics.

The second effect is usually more unpleasant than serious. Nausea or vomiting are common, especially following upon the administration of a narcotic analgesic. According to one report about 40 per cent of patients experience nausea and up to 20 per cent actually vomit after an injection of morphine. Although it is often said that pethidine is less likely to cause nausea and vomiting than morphine it is doubtful if this statement is true. Nausea and vomiting are due to the action of the drug on the vomiting centre in the brain and not usually to a direct action on the gut. The phenothiazine derivatives are often effective against this type of vomiting and so is the antihistaminic cyclizine. A combined injection of cyclizine 50 mg and morphine 10 mg is available as Cyclimorph. Droperidol (Droleptan) and haloperidol (Serenace) are other effective anti-emetics.

Effect on labour

Text books are full of half-truths about the effect of analgesics and sedatives on progress in labour. It is often stated that these drugs diminish uterine activity and prolong labour. A large dose of morphine may occasionally depress uterine contractions when given before labour is properly established. A well-timed dose of a narcotic analgesic will not inhibit the contractions of established labour. Indeed a judicious dose of morphine or pethidine will sometimes accelerate progress in labour, perhaps by relieving the inhibitory effect of pain and anxiety.

The narcotic antagonists

Nalorphine (Lethidrone, Nalline) and levallorphan (Lorfan) were the two specific antagonists to the narcotic analgesics in general use until recently. These two antagonists are derivatives of morphine and a morphine-like drug levorphan (Dromoran). Naloxone (Narcan) is a new narcotic antagonist and is a derivative of oxymorphone (Numorphan). Naloxone is now the antagonist of choice because it is itself completely free of any morphine-like action.

The subject of the narcotic antagonists is complex and in some respects controversial. The following fundamentals are generally agreed.

1. When nalorphine, levallorphan or naloxone is administered to a patient who has respiratory depression due to one of the narcotic analgesics then there will be a rapid and substantial increase in the rate and depth of respiration. To a lesser extent the other signs of narcotic overdose will be reversed. The level of consciousness will be raised, hypotension will be partly reversed and the analgesic action of the narcotic will be lessened.

2. The narcotic antagonists are specific antagonists. They act only against morphine, pethidine and the various other opiate and synthetic narcotic analgesics. They do not antagonise the effects of an overdose of barbiturates, phenothiazine derivates or general anaesthetics. Naloxone is a specific antagonist to pentazocine.

3. When administered to a patient who is not suffering from depression due to one of the narcotic analgesics, nalorphine and levallorphan will themselves act as narcotics. This is because these antagonists are chemical relations of morphine. Fortunately, if the antagonist naloxone is used, there will be no unwanted narcotic action and it is this which makes naloxone the preferred narcotic antagonist.

The accurage diagnosis of the cause of respiratory depression is essential, otherwise the situation may be worsened. If the depression is in fact due to a drug other than a narcotic analgesic, or is not due to any drug, then nalorphine and levallorphan will aggravate the depression by acting as a narcotic. In such circumstances the administration of naloxone should be harmless.

The narcotic antagonists readily cross the placental barrier and if given intravenously to the mother shortly before delivery they will prevent narcotic-induced respiratory depression in the newborn. The antagonists may also be administered to the infant at birth and this is the preferred method. It is notoriously difficult to predict whether or not an infant will suffer from the effects of narcotic analgesics given to the mother during labour and it is more logical to treat the infant when necessary. The only satisfactory route of administration to the newborn is by the umbilical vein. The effects of an intramuscular injection are too long delayed.

Suggested doses of narcotic antagonists are as shown in Table 1.

Table 1 Doses of narcotic antagonists

For the mother:	Nalorphine (Nalline, Lethidrone)	5 mg to 10 mg
	Levallorphan (Lorfan)	0.5 mg to 1 mg
	Naloxone (Narcan)	0.4 mg to 0.8 mg
For the newborn:	Nalorphine (Nalline, Lethidrone)	0.5 mg to 1 mg
	Levallorphan (Lorfan)	0.05 mg to 0.1 mg
	Naloxone (Narcan)	0.04 mg to 0.08 mg
	(There is a neonatal solution of naloxone)	

The above doses may be expected to reverse the effects of approximately 10 mg morphine or 100 mg pethidine. Larger doses of narcotic analgesic may require larger doses of antagonist for the complete reversal of depression. Ideally the dose of the antagonist should be balanced or titrated against the dose of the narcotic analgesic.

The decision to administer nalorphine or levallorphan to a particular infant requires good judgement. The total dose of narcotic analgesics given to the mother should be assessed and it should be remembered that narcotic-induced respiratory depression is likely to be greatest between one and a half and two hours after the administration of the drug. Naloxone being devoid of depressant effects may safely be given, even although the cause of the neonatal depression is in doubt.

Pethilorfan

It is on the subject of pre-mixed solutions of narcotic and antagonist that most controversy arises. Pethilorfan is a mixture of pethidine 100 mg with levallorphan (Lorfan) 1.25 mg in a 2 ml ampoule and is approved for use by midwives. The claim for Pethilorfan is analgesia without respiratory depression. Were this claim to be substantiated then the greatest single problem of analgesic therapy would have been solved. Unfortunately a careful assessment of the evidence suggests quite strongly that Pethilorfan cannot be relied upon to produce analgesia without depressing respiration.

The evidence is often contradictory and most of the favourable claims seem to have been based on enthusiasm rather than on controlled trials and statistical analyses. At least one well-conducted investigation has shown that Pethilorfan actually caused more respiratory depression than pethidine! It has also been suggested that the analgesic action of Pethilorfan is less than that of pethidine. Combinations of pethidine and naloxone have recently been found to produce less pain relief than pethidine alone. There is no doubt that levallorphan, nalorphine and naloxone are effective antagonists when given in the presence of existing narcotic-induced depression, it is the value of the simultaneous prophylactic administration of narcotic and antagonist which is in doubt. Pethilorfan is now much less frequently used and a growing body of opinion favours the use of a narcotic analgesic during labour and the administration of an antagonist to the infant who is born with narcotic-induced respiratory depression. It is my opinion that Pethilorfan should no longer be used.

The treatment of pain with drugs

The objective of all treatment in pregnancy is the delivery of a healthy child from a healthy and emotionally satisfied mother. The proper management of pain in labour plays an important part in achieving emotional satisfaction and can also contribute to the physical well-being of mother and child. Many women who view motherhood with joy may yet be terrified of labour and the pain which they associate with the birth process. The midwife can do much to reassure the patient by imparting knowledge and by her sympathetic but firm manner.

Nevertheless, the majority of patients experience pain in labour and require analgesia, whether by drugs or other means. In the past women have sometimes deliberately avoided any subsequent pregnancy because of the memory of intolerable pain and distress suffered during a first prolonged labour. The effects of such a decision on the emotional stability and the marriages of these women must have been profound.

The rational choice of a drug or a combination of drugs can only be made after due consideration of the needs of the individual patient and the actions of the available drugs. For example it is folly to attempt to treat anxiety which is due mainly to pain by administering a sedative or tranquillising drug unless an analgesic is also administered. Sometimes the relief of pain by an injection of pethidine will abolish anxiety and an anxiety-relieving drug is unnecessary.

The precise cause of pain in labour is uncertain. Uterine contractions during late pregnancy are painless. Is it dilatation of the cervix, ischaemia of the uterine muscle or merely the greater intensity of the contractions which makes them painful? Whatever the explanation, pain is the indication for analgesia, regardless of the dilatation of the cervix. Pain is experienced in the cutaneous distribution of the eleventh and twelfth thoracic and first lumbar nerves, because these are the nerves which transmit painful sensations from the uterus. The pain of uterine contractions is thus a type of referred pain.

It may be argued that both pain and anxiety are present in nearly all women during labour. Upon this belief is based the popular practice of administering a tranquilliser such as promazine (Sparine) and an analgesic such as pethidine routinely in labour. Although there is experimental evidence that certain phenothiazine derivatives and barbiturates can antagonise the analgesic action of pethidine, clinical experience confirms the value of combinations such as pethidine and promazine for patients who are both anxious and in pain. When labour is not yet established and painful but anxiety is a feature, a sedative or tranquilliser may be administered alone. Again a hypnotic drug may permit a few hours of valuable sleep for a patient in early labour. The midwife can prescribe chloral hydrate, triclofos or Welldorm tablets in sedative or hypnotic doses.

None of the narcotic analgesics will give complete relief of pain to all patients when given in safe doses. In hospital practice the percentage of patients who do not obtain adequate pain relief from drugs and inhalational methods is disappointingly high. In a survey conducted in Sheffield 40 per cent of patients were dissatisfied with the analgesia provided by liberal doses of narcotic analgesics and by inhalational methods. A recent report from the Hammersmith Hospital indicated that only 22 per cent of patients received satisfactory analgesia from pethidine alone and 48 per cent obtained no relief whatsoever from this drug. Complete analgesia was never obtained. Where possible other methods of pain relief such as epidural analgesia should be available to supplement drug therapy during labour. Unfortunately epidural analgesia is often unavailable outside teaching hospitals and the best possible use must be made of the methods available to obstetricians and midwives.

Because it is doubtful if any one narcotic analgesic gives significantly better pain relief or significantly less respiratory depression in equi-analgesic doses, it is not necessary to employ a whole pharmacopoeia of analgesic drugs. From a small number of carefully chosen drugs one can achieve certain effects which are appropriate for each patient. One may wish to utilise the sedative properties of morphine, the euphoriant action of diamorphine (heroin) or the relative absence of these effects when pethidine is used.

In the management of pain it is a good principle to give an effective dose of analgesic drug at the outset and thereafter to maintain analgesia by subsequent smaller doses. In this way pain is more rapidly and effectively relieved and the patient's faith in the drug and in her attendants is not destroyed. The primary indication for the administration of an analgesic to a woman in labour is pain. This is surely obvious and yet there are those who prescribe analgesics according to the extent of dilatation of the cervix and would withhold drugs because the cervix is not yet 4 cm dilated or whatever other figure may be selected. The practice of prescribing analgesics solely according to cervical dilatation is mentioned only to condemn it.

In Fig. 1 there is a schematic representation of the times in labour during which the various methods of analgesia may be

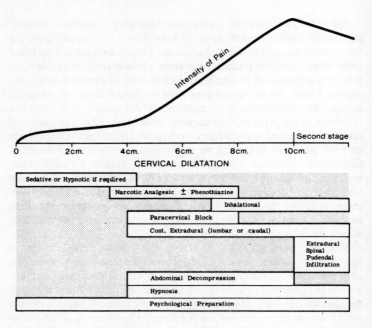

Fig 1 A representation of the timing of various methods of analgesia in relation to pain and to cervical dilatation. Pain rather than cervical dilatation is the indication for analgesia.

used. Pain is shown as being maximal at 9 to 10 cm dilatation, but pain rather than cervical dilatation is the indication for analgesia. There is no distinction made between primigravidae and multigravidae in this diagram. Pethidine acts until delivery although its administration will have ceased before this. Inhalational analgesia may be commenced before 8 cm dilatation. Although pudendal, epidural and spinal blocks are not usually intitiated in the second stage for spontaneous vertex deliveries in the United Kingdom, it should be remembered that the forceps delivery rate exceeds 20 per cent in many hospitals and so there is a definite place for these techniques in the second stage of labour.

The observer can only assess the patient's response to pain and cannot accurately assess the pain itself. The stoical woman who suppresses her natural responses to pain appears to have little pain, while the patient who cries out with every uterine contraction gives the appearance of suffering great pain. In the final analysis the patient must be the judge of the severity of her pain and of the effectiveness of analgesic therapy.

There is no place for subcutaneous injections of analgesics in labour because absorption is too slow and too erratic. Injections should normally be given intramuscularly. Where pain relief is urgent an intravenous injection of pethidine can be useful, but must be given by a doctor and will result in free placental transfer of pethidine. Towards the end of the first stage of labour when pain is most intense, intramuscular injections are relatively ineffective. An intravenous injection of up to 50 mg of pethidine should be given slowly over 5 to 10 minutes and the drug should be diluted before injection. The risk of hypotension and vomiting in the mother and respiratory depression in the newborn is increased when intravenous injections of narcotic analgesics are given. An apparatus has been described which permits the self-administration of a fixed dose of pethidine intravenously at intervals. There is a minimum interval between doses and the possibility of serious overdose is further reduced by the need to pass a test of reaction time before each injection. Mothers found the method acceptable and it is said to be suitable for use by midwives under supervision (Evans et al, (1976) Lancet, i, 17). The placental transfer of pethidine would be extensive with this technique. An alternative to intravenous analgesia late in the first stage is, of course, inhalational analgesia.

A slow, continuous intravenous infusion of a very dilute solution of an analgesic is a fairly efficient and controllable method of pain relief which could, with benefit, be more extensively used. Side-effects are much less likely to occur than after a single intravenous injection. The addition of 200 mg of pethidine to 500 ml of infusion fluid allows finger-tip control of analgesia by altering the drip rate to meet the patient's analgesic requirements. Electronic drip counters and motor driven syringes are useful but inessential refinements in the control of continuous intravenous analgesic therapy. I believe that the skilful use of intravenous infusions of analgesic drugs can give better pain relief than is sometimes obtained with intramuscular injections of the same drugs. This sort of therapy does not require the skills of a specialist anaesthetist which are often lacking when abnormally painful labour might otherwise have been managed under epidural analgesia, but does require medical supervision. Unfortunately intravenous infusions of analgesic drugs are associated with free placental transfer and a high risk of neonatal depression.

Lastly, there are extraneous factors whose importance must be recalled. The labour room should be attractively decorated and furnished and the 'hospital' atmosphere should be kept to a minimum in a normal labour. The presence of the husband should be encouraged, if the patient and her husband wish this. It is helpful if the patient has already become acquainted with her attendant midwife and doctor during her pregnancy. In domiciliary midwifery the familiar surroundings and attendants, together with the careful selection of patients for their normality and usually their multiparity, all contribute to the relatively easy and painless labours characteristic of many home confinements. To a considerable extent these features are also to be found in the general practitioner maternity unit.

Prescribing by midwives

A practising midwife is authorised to prescribe certain sedative, hypnotic and analgesic drugs, subject to the provisions of the relevant Misuse of Drugs Regulations and Central Midwives Boards' rules. The Central Midwives Boards have ruled that: 'A practising midwife must not on her own responsibility use any drug, including an analgesic unless in the course of her training, whether before or after enrolment she has been thoroughly instructed in its use and is familiar with its dosage and methods of administration or application.'

The drugs which a practising midwife may prescribe, subject to the foregoing provisions are:

Chloral hydrate, triclofos (Tricloryl), dichlorphenazone (Welldorm), tincture of opium, pethidine and Pethilorfan, pentazocine and promazine.

In the case of pethidine and Pethilorfan the midwife must observe the provisions of the Misuse of Drugs Regulations applicable to midwives. She must keep a drug book in which she records the quantities of pethidine and Pethilorfan supplied to her and the quanitites administered by her together with the name and address of the patient and the date of administration. A midwife in domiciliary practice may be supplied with pethidine under the Misuse of Drugs Regulations (1973), Part II, section 11 and the Misuse of Drugs (Amendment) Regulations 1974, paragraph 4. The midwife obtains a supply order signed by an 'appropriate medical officer' who is either a doctor authorised by the local supervising authority (the Health Board) or a person appointed by the Health Board to exercise supervision over certified midwives. The supply order should state the total quantity to be supplied and the purpose for which it is required. Dangerous drugs must be kept in a locked receptacle when not in use (a locked motor car does not meet the requirements of the Regulations).

The dose of pethidine which a domiciliary midwife may prescribe is not specified by the C. M. B. It is, however, widely held that she should not administer more than 200 mg to one patient and that she should not give more than 100 mg in one injection. This seems prudent advice. The maximum dose is laid down by the supervising authority. The midwife should remain with any patient to whom she has given pethidine. At the present time the midwife who works in hospital is not normally allowed to prescribe pethidine. Nevertheless the Aiken Report (*Control of Dangerous Drugs and Poisons in Hospitals* H. M. S. O. 1958), while acknowledging that pethidine is usually prescribed by a doctor and that there should be a single source of supply of all drugs in a hospital, recommended that measures be taken to ensure that a midwife could administer pethidine on her own initiative, in the absence of a doctor. The details of the procedure for each hospital should be agreed between the midwives and doctors and should then be displayed in the maternity unit.

Drug interactions

The possibility of dangerous and even fatal reactions occurring after the administration of analgesic or sedative drugs must be known to everyone who uses these drugs. Ever growing numbers of patients regularly take medicaments in an effort to combat the stresses of modern living and a number of the drugs used in psychiatric practice are capable of interacting with narcotic analgesics and causing disastrous effects upon the patient. Unless a careful enquiry is made, those attending the patient in labour may be unaware that the woman is under treatment with drugs. It is recommended that every patient be asked about treatment with drugs on admission to hospital or when first seen in pregnancy. It should be remembered that some patients will be reluctant to admit to undergoing psychiatric treatment, whether by a general practitioner or a psychiatrist.

Any previously administered sedative, hypnotic or tranquillising drug will exaggerate the effects of narcotic analgesics, tranquillisers and sedatives given during labour. The greatest danger lies in the administration of pethidine, morphine and probably any of the other narcotic analgesics to a patient already under treatment with one of the monoamine oxidase inhibitors. These drugs are used in the treatment of depressive states and the commoner monoamine oxidase inhibitors include the following:

Isocarboxazid (Marplan)	Phenelzine (Nardil)
Mebanazine (Actomol)	Nialamide (Niamid)
Pheniprazine (Cavodil)	Tranylcypromine (Parnate and
Phenoxypropazine (Drazine)	a constituent of Parstelin)
Pargyline (Eutonyl)	Pivhydrazine (Tersavid)
Iproniazid (Marsilid)	Etryptamine (Monase)

The administration of a narcotic analgesic to a patient who has taken a monoamine oxidase inhibitor may produce prolonged and deep coma with profound respiratory depression and hypotension and this type of drug interaction could prove fatal for the mother or her infant. Intravenous hydrocortisone may be useful in treating this type of reaction. Morphine, pethidine and allied analgesics should not be given to patients who are being treated with a monoamine oxidase inhibitor. An alternative method of pain relief should be used. Fortunately monoamine oxidase inhibitors are now less frequently prescribed.

Certain other forms of therapy may cause serious effects

during labour. Previous treatment with hypotensive agents (including those used in pre-eclampsia) may occasionally lead to a severe fall in blood pressure when sedatives or analgesics are given during labour. Current or recent treatment with corticosteroids may occasionally be associated with collapse and hypotension during labour. The administration of epidural or spinal analgesia to a patient who has received analgesic, sedative or tranquillising drugs may result in an excessive fall in blood pressure.

4. Individual Sedatives, Analgesics and Tranquillisers

This chapter has two objectives. The first is to provide the midwife with information about the properties, doses and actions of the drugs which she can administer on her own responsibility. The second objective is to make available to the midwife a readily accessible source of reference to other sedatives, analgesics and tranquillisers which are used in the management of normal and abnormal labour, but which are prescribed by a doctor. It is obviously essential that the midwife must have a sound knowledge of the drugs which she can administer on her own authority. It is also desirable that she should have an understanding of the drugs which are prescribed by the doctor to patients under her care. It is not intended that the midwife should memorise detailed information about all the drugs which may be used in labour. It is more important to understand the general principles outlined in Chapter 3.

Drugs prescribed by a midwife

Until recently, old-fashioned preparations of limited value (e.g. potassium bromide and Dover's powder) were prescribable by midwives and their removal from the list of approved drugs is welcomed. It is my opinion that tincture of opium should be allowed to share the fate of Dover's powder.

Chloral hydrate, triclofos and dichlorphenazone

These three drugs are broken down in the body to the same substance (trichlorethanol) and this is the active sedative and hypnotic agent. Consequently the sedative and hypnotic effect of the three parent drugs is identical. The differences are those of palatability and gastric side-effects. Syrup of chloral has an unpleasant taste and may irritate the stomach causing nausea and vomiting. Triclofos (Tricloryl) or Welldorm (chloral hydrate and

Table 2 Drugs which a midwife may prescribe and administer on her own responsibility to a woman in labour.

Sedatives, hypnotics and tranquillisers

	Recommended dose	Other names
Chloral hydrate	0.5 g to 2 g	Chloral mixture or syrup, Somnos elixir and capsules, Somilan, Valibrom, Hydratine.
Triclofos	0.5 g to 1 g	Tricloryl syrup and tablets.
Dichlorphenazone tablets (each contains chloral hydrate 0.65 g and phenazone 1.3 g)	1 or 2 tablets	Welldorm.
Promazine hydrochloride	25 mg to 50 mg	Sparine, tablets or injection.
Tincture of opium	0.5 ml to 1 ml	*tinct. opii.* *Laudanum.*

Analgesics

Pethidine	100 mg to 150 mg	Demerol.
Pethilorfan (2 ml contains 100 mg pethidine and 1.25 mg levallorphan)	100 mg to 150 mg	
Pentazocine	40 mg to 60 mg	Fortral.

A midwife may also prescribe ergometrine and oxytocin and administer prostaglandins.

dichlorphenazone) tablets are less likely to cause gastric irritation and are preferred for adult patients.

These drugs are very safe and in normal dosage (see Table 2) they should not affect cardiac or respiratory function. The smaller doses are useful as sedatives in early labour. The larger doses will promote sleep. If pain is present an analgesic drug must also be given because these drugs have no analgesic action.

Tincture of opium. (Tinct. opii, laudanum)

This preparation contains about 1 per cent of morphine and also contains 20 or more other alkaloids of opium. Its action is therefore somewhat unpredictable and can be expected to vary according to the proportions of the various constituent alkaloids. Tincture of opium has sedative and mild analgesic properties.

The midwife who wishes to prescribe a sedative or hypnotic drug is advised to use triclofos or Welldorm tablets.

Pethidine (meperidine, demerol)

Pethidine is a synthetic narcotic with a powerful analgesic action. In equi-analgesic doses the sedative action of pethidine is less than that of morphine. The analgesic effects of 100 mg pethidine are approximately the same as those of 10 mg morphine. Pethidine is particularly effective against pain of visceral origin, such as biliary and renal colic and of course the pain of labour. Pethidine begins to act about 20 minutes after an intramuscular injection and two minutes after an intravenous injection. Intramuscular injections may be required at intervals of two to four hours during labour.

Pethidine is a drug of addiction. The possibility of producing addiction by administering pethidine to a normal woman in labour is negligible. A woman who is already addicted to other drugs might conceivably become addicted to pethidine given in labour. Midwives who have access to pethidine have from time to time become addicts.

Pethidine has important side-effects on various body systems.

Respiratory system

Pethidine depresses respiration. Because pethidine freely crosses the placental barrier it may cause neonatal respiratory depression. Commonly the blood level of pethidine in the infant is about 70 per cent of the maternal level. The depressant effect of pethidine on neonatal respiration is the greatest danger of this drug in midwifery. Established respiratory depression can be treated with nalorphine (Lethidrone), levallorphan (Lorfan), or naloxone (Narcan). The mother's pain may stimulate her respirations and counteract the depressant effect of pethidine, but of course this does nothing to counteract depression in the newborn. The narcotic antagonists are discussed on page 20.

Cardiovascular system

Blood pressure is usually unaffected while the patient remains in bed, but may fall suddenly if she sits or stands (orthostatic hypotension). Single intravenous injections are liable to cause hypotension. Combinations of pethidine and a phenothiazine derivative or a barbiturate may lower the blood pressure.

The uterus

Pethidine does not affect the uterine contractions of established, normal labour. In an inco-ordinate labour, the administration of pethidine may be followed by more rapid dilatation of the cervical os. This beneficial effect is probably due to the release of muscular tension following upon the relief of pain, rather than to any direct anti-spasmodic action of pethidine on the uterus.

Alimentary system

Pethidine often causes nausea and occasionally causes vomiting. Gastric emptying may be delayed. Phenothiazine derivatives or cyclizine may be used in the treatment of troublesome nausea and vomiting. Droperidol (Droleptan) is a powerful anti-emetic.

The liver

Pethidine is broken down in the liver and the break down products are excreted in the urine. The hormonal changes in pregnancy may modify the breakdown of pethidine. In severe liver disease the destruction of pethidine may be impaired and its action may be prolonged and intensified.

Pethidine is often given along with phenothiazine derivatives such as promethazine (Phenergan) and promazine (Sparine) in

25 mg or 50 mg doses. In these circumstances the dose of pethidine should be reduced because the sedative and hypotensive effects of these drug combinations are greater than those of pethidine alone.

Warning

Serious reactions, including coma, profound hypotension and respiratory depression may occur when pethidine is given to patients under treatment with monoamine oxidase inhibitors (see note on Drug Interactions on page 30).

Pethilorfan

This is a combination of 100 mg pethidine and 1.25 mg. levallorphan (Lorfan) in 2 ml of solution. Pethilorfan has been discussed at some length on page 23 and the reasons for not recommending this drug have been detailed. It is probable that Pethilorfan is a weaker analgesic than pethidine and that respiratory depression is not in fact prevented.

Pentazocine (Fortral)

This relatively new synthetic analgesic is not an opium derivative. An important advantage of pentazocine is that it does not cause serious addiction even after repeated administration and the drug is not subject to the Misuse of Drugs Regulations. Pentazocine 40 mg produces a comparable degree of analgesia and respiratory depression to 100 mg pethidine. Respiratory depression due to pentazocine is not reversible by nalorphine and levallorphan but may be reversed by naloxon. Pentazocine crosses the placental barrier.

In one recent study 40 mg pentazocine was as effective an analgesic in labour as 100 mg pethidine and the incidence of nausea and vomiting was less with pentazocine. Many patients will not obtain satisfactory relief of pain unless 60 mg pentazocine is given. Pentazocine may establish a place for itself in midwifery, mainly because its use is very unlikely to lead to addiction and it is otherwise fairly comparable to pethidine. The C. M. B. has recently approved the use of pentazocine by midwives. Pentazocine may be useful for patients who experience nausea or vomiting with opiate analgesics.

Drugs prescribed by a doctor

Sedatives and tranquillisers

Almost every known sedative and tranquilliser must have been used during labour at some time or other. Only a few of the more popular and representative drugs will be considered and even these are listed mainly for reference. The midwife need only learn the details of the pharmacology of those drugs which are in use in her own hospital or practice.

The barbiturates.

The medium and short acting barbiturates such as pentobarbitone (Nembutal), amylobarbitone (Amytal), butobarbitone (Soneryl) and quinalbarbitone (Seconal) are sedative and hypnotic drugs whose action lasts for four to six hours. The sedative dose of these drugs is 30 mg to 60 mg. A hypnotic effect may be obtained after a dose of 100 mg to 200 mg.

The barbiturates have no analgesic action but may modify the patient's response to her pain. If pain is not relieved by the simultaneous administration of an analgesic the patient may lose her self control and become disorientated and difficult to manage.

Side-effects include hypotension and respiratory depression after large doses. Placental transfer is free and the breakdown and elimination of these drugs by the fetus and newborn is slow. The newborn infant may take three or four days to eliminate barbiturates from its body and may be sluggish and drowsy at birth. There is no effective antidote to the barbiturates. For these reasons the barbiturates are now seldom prescribed during labour. They are still occasionally used for their sedative and anticonvulsant action in pre-eclampsia and they have a mild hypotensive effect in hypertensive patients. Phenobarbitone (Gardenal) is an anticonvulsant drug for the prevention of eclampsia. Better and safer sedatives and anticonvulsants are available.

Phenothiazine derivatives

The phenothiazine derivatives are known as tranquillisers or ataractics and are often prescribed in labour. They relieve or reduce anxiety without inducing drowsiness to the extent which may occur with the older-established sedative drugs.

The phenothiazines also have anti-emetic and anti-histamine actions. They may cause hypotension after intravenous administration but this effect is rarely seen after an intramuscular injection. The phenothiazine derivatives are usually given along with pethidine and although the phenothiazine derivatives are not themselves analgesic drugs they may reduce the need for analgesics. Phenothiazines may have a rather longer duration of action than pethidine and so a second injection of pethidine may not require a concomitant injection of phenothiazine. The phenothiazines do not depress respiration in the doses used in labour and in practice are safe and useful drugs. Uterine contractions are not inhibited. The phenothiazine derivatives cross the placental barrier but experience suggests that they do not significantly affect the newborn infant. Amnesia sometimes occurs after the administration of the phenothiazine derivatives.

The two phenothiazine derivatives in general use are promazine (Sparine) and promethazine (Phenergan). They are given by intramuscular injection in doses of 25 mg or 50 mg. When pethidine is given at the same time it is customary to reduce the dose of the analgesic drug by about one third. Promazine may cause fetal and maternal tachycardia. Chlorpromazine (Largactil) is now rarely used because the incidence of side-effects is relatively high. Promazine has recently been approved by the C. M. B. for use by midwives. The phenothiazines are now less often prescribed in labour.

Nitrazepam (Mogadon). This rapidly acting hynotic is much safer than the barbiturates if an overdose is taken and recovery from a normal hynotic dose is relatively free from hang-over. Where a simple hypnotic is required then nitrazepam 5 mg or 10 mg is preferable to a barbiturate.

Hyoscine (Scopolamine). Hyoscine has been used for many years as a sedative in labour. Hyoscine sometimes causes amnesia for the events of labour and was formerly used along with morphine to induce twilight sleep. Hyoscine 0.4 mg is combined with a narcotic analgesic but has been less frequently used since the introduction of the phenothiazine derivatives and diazepam.

Diazepam (Valium). This interesting new drug has been used in obstetrics as a tranquilliser and as an anticonvulsant. It is not an analgesic, and an analgesic such as pethidine should also be given in active labour. Placental transfer occurs but it has been claimed that diazepam does not depress the newborn. Amnesia sometimes follows its administration. Diazepam is given by intramuscular injection in a dose of 20 mg to 40 mg and may also be given intravenously, in 5 mg to 10 mg doses. It has been claimed that the use of diazepam reduces the dose of pethidine required for the satisfactory relief of pain. Diazepam must not be mixed with other drugs in the same syringe. The powerful anti-convulsant action of diazepam has been utilised in the prevention and treatment of eclampsia, epilepsy and other convulsant states. It has been suggested that diazepam may occasionally cause hypothermia and hypotonia in the newborn and that in the severely jaundiced infant there may be an increased liability to kernicterus. Nevertheless the great majority of infants appear to be unaffected. It is recommended that if diazepam is used in labour then the total dose should not exceed 40 mg. In the treatment of convulsive states it may be necessary and justifiable to exceed this dose. Diazepam does not lower the blood pressure.

Droperidol (Droleptan). This drug, like its relative haloperidol (Serenace) is a neuroleptic and can produce a state of calmness sometimes associated with feelings of indifference and detachment. Occasionally these feelings may distress the patient. Droperidol and haloperidol have a strong anti-emetic action. Occasionally extra-pyramidal side effects may follow their administration and these effects may not develop for up to 24 hours. Respiratory depression and hypotension are rare. Droperidol is given by intramuscular injection in doses of 5 mg to 10 mg and it may also be given intravenously in smaller doses. If pain is present an analgesic should also be given.

Chlormethiazole (Heminevrin). This drug has sedative, hypnotic and anticonvulsant actions and has been favourably reported on in the management of pre-eclampsia and eclampsia. It may be given orally in the form of 500 mg capsules. During labour a continuous infusion of 0.8 per cent chlormethiazole is used to produce a hypnotic and anticonvulsant effect. Hypotension and analgesia must be obtained by other means, so that chlormethiazole is then used as part of a regime of balanced therapy for patients with pre-eclampsia who are in labour. There should be no question of inducing basal narcosis with the chlormethiazole infusion and the patient should remain capable of rational conversation and an infusion rate of about 60 drops per minute for 10 minutes, followed by a maintenance rate of about 20 drops per minute is usually satisfactory. Chlormethiazole infusions have been successfully combined with epidural analgesia in the Queen Mother's Hospital, Glasgow. Alternatively the combination of chlormethiazole, pethidine and protoveratrine (Puroverine) advocated by the Aberdeen workers may be used to obtain sedation, analgesia, hypotension and an anticonvulsant effect. Chlormethiazole infusions have been used to obliterate all conscious memory of labour in the occasional patient for whom this has been considered desirable. Two 500 mg capsules have been used as a safe sedative in normal labour.

Bromethol (tribromethanol, Avertin). Bromethol is a basal narcotic which is administered rectally. Bromethol depresses the functions of all parts of the central nervous system and causes unconsciousness, hypotension and respiratory depression. Liver damage may occur. Bromethol has no analgesic action.

Bromethol is used in the management of severe pre-eclampsia and eclampsia, where despite its dangers it can effectively lower the blood pressure and prevent or abolish convulsions. Nevertheless, it is my belief that there are now safer and equally, if not more effective methods of managing impending or actual eclampsia.

Bromethol is given in a dose of 80 mg to 100 mg per kg of body weight (up to 120 mg per kg has been used). Bromethol is available as Avertin solution containing 1g in each 1 ml. Before administering the drug the concentrated Avertin solution must be diluted with 40 parts of distilled water to one part of Avertin solution. The distilled water must be at a temperature of between 32°C (90°F) and 40°C (104°F). The diluted Avertin must be tested for impurities by the addition of a few drops of Congo red to about 5 ml of the Avertin solution. A red colour indicates that the mixture is safe for use. A blue colour means that the mixture must on no account be used. The calculated dose is run into the rectum over a period of 5 to 10 minutes. The muscular effort sometimes associated with a uterine contraction may result in the loss of bromethol solution from the rectum and absorption from the rectum is rather uncertain. If the buttocks are pressed together during and after the administration then loss of solution is less likely.

Apart from the time required to prepare and administer bromethol and the possibility of loss or incomplete absorption from the rectum the major problem of bromethol therapy is that the patient often loses consciousness, sometimes for several hours and is therefore liable to develop the well-recognised complications of the unconscious state. She may aspirate stomach contents into her lungs and may develop infection and pulmonary collapse. The patient who has received a full dose of bromethol should be nursed as an unconscious patient. She must be attended to constantly and should be nursed on her side and turned on to the opposite side at two hourly intervals. Apparatus for tracheal and pharyngeal suction should be available.

'Lytic cocktail'. This term refers to any of various mixtures of phenothiazine derivatives and pethidine for intravenous administration. For example, a mixture of chlorpromazine (Largactil) 50 mg, promethazine (Phenergan) 50 mg and pethidine 100 mg may be diluted and given slowly intravenously until a state of sedation, tranquility and analgesia (ataralgesia) is produced. The 'lytic cocktail' is used in the treatment of eclampsia and severe pre-eclampsia. In these conditions a useful hypotensive action can be obtained but the prevention of convulsions is less certain. The 'lytic cocktail' has been used in conjunction with regional analgesia for forceps delivery, breech delivery and Caesarean section.

Magnesium sulphate. Magnesium sulphate has a depressant action on the central and peripheral nervous systems and is still occasionally used in the treatment of eclampsia. The drug has anticonvulsant, sedative and hypotensive effects and may reduce cerebral oedema. The results of magnesium sulphate therapy appear to be less satisfactory than those obtained with bromethol, the 'lytic cocktail' or chlormethiazole. Magnesium sulphate may be given intravenously (up to 20 ml of a 20 per cent solution) or it may be given per rectum. Magnesium sulphate is more extensively used in the U.S.A. and one regime used in treating eclampsia consists of two separate deep intramuscular injections of 10 ml of a 50 per cent aqueous solution, followed by single injections of 10 ml at intervals of 4 to 6 hours. The injections are painful. Respiratory depression may occur and regular estimations of the serum magnesium concentration are advisable. The slow intravenous injection of one gram of calcium gluconate may be used in the treatment of magnesium intoxication.

Paraldehyde. Paraldehyde is no longer used as a sedative during normal labour, but is still occasionally used in pre-eclampsia, eclampsia and delirious states as a sedative and anticonvulsant. It is given by intravenous, intramuscular or rectal injection. A dose of 10 ml to 15 ml may be given by intravenous or intramuscular injection. A glass syringe should be used because paraldehyde dissolves plastic. The dose for rectal infusion is 0.5 ml per kg body weight. Intramuscular injections are painful and irritant and not more than 5 ml should be injected at one site. There are better drugs available for the management of eclampsia.

Narcotic Analgesics

Morphine. Morphine is a most valuable drug in labour. Seldom used routinely, morphine in the opinion of many experienced obstetricians is superior to pethidine when labour is prolonged and painful and delivery is not anticipated for at least three or four hours. Morphine is sometimes given as the first analgesic drug to the primigravida who is in early but painful labour and it is useful in inco-ordinate labour and in any abnormally painful labour. When the occiput is in the posterior position labour is often more protracted and more painful and morphine is of great value. Morphine and allied compounds are less frequently needed when labour is accelerated or augmented with oxytocin.

Morphine is no better an analgesic than pethidine in equipotent doses but the sedative and hypnotic properties exceed those of pethidine and the ability of morphine to relieve the anxiety inevitably associated with a prolonged labour is well recognised. The price to be paid for the benefits of morphine includes a predisposition to respiratory depression in the mother and the newborn, a slight risk of maternal hypotension and a high incidence of nausea and vomiting. The uterine contractions of established labour are unaffected and in inco-ordinate uterine action a more normal type of uterine action may follow the administration of morphine.

The respiratory depressant action of morphine and all the narcotic analgesics can be reversed by the narcotic antagonists nalorphine, levallorphan and naloxone. Even so, it is usually advised that morphine should not be given within three to four hours of anticipated delivery.

The usual dose of morphine is 15 mg, although a dose of 10 mg may be sufficient and is less likely to produce unpleasant side effects.

Papaveretum (Omnopon, Pantopon, Alopon). This preparation contains 50 per cent of morphine together with various other alkaloids of opium. Thus the usual 20 mg dose of papaveretum contains 10 mg morphine. In practice the morphine content of 20 mg papaveretum is more nearly equivalent in effect to 15 mg morphine sulphate. (This is because the morphine in papaveretum is anhydrous and an injection of morphine sulphate contains water molecules.) An injection of papaveretum will have the effects of nearly 15 mg of morphine and the effects of the other constituent alkaloids of opium. Hyoscine 0.4 mg is sometimes given along with papaveretum when the sedative action will be enhanced and amnesia may be produced. It has been claimed that the incidence of nausea and vomiting is less after papaveretum and hyoscine (Omnopon and Scopolamine) than after morphine.

Diamorphine (heroin, diacetylmorphine). Diamorphine is a powerful narcotic analgesic which induces an intense feeling of euphoria and well-being usually without much drowsiness. It is given in doses of 5 mg to 7.5 mg and is particularly valuable for the anxious primigravida in early labour. Diamorphine carries a high risk of addiction even after a few doses, but there should be no risk attached to a single injection in a patient who is not prone to drug addiction. Diamorphine is no longer prescribable in the U.S.A. but many British doctors believe that this drug has a small but valuable role in treating pain and anxiety. Diamorphine is antagonised by nalorphine, levallorphan and naloxone.

Oxymorphone (Numorphan). Oxymorphone is a synthetic

morphine derivative which is administered in doses of 1 mg to 1.5 mg. Oxymorphone has been claimed to cause less nausea and vomiting than morphine but has no other confirmed advantages over the parent drug. Respiratory depression is probably just as great in equi-analgesic doses and can be reversed by narcotic antagonists.

Methadone (Physeptone, amidone). Methadone is a synthetic analgesic and its dose is from 5 mg to 10 mg. The effects and side effects of methadone are similar to those of the other narcotic analgesics and respiratory depression is reversible by nalorphine levallorphan and naloxone.

Alphaprodine (Nisentil). This is a synthetic analgesic related to pethidine and is administered in doses of from 30 mg to 60 mg. Alphaprodine is similar in action to pethidine and does not appear to have any important advantages. The narcotic antagonists are effective.

Dihydrocodeine (DF 118). This is a derivative of codeine with an analgesic potency greater than codeine but less than pethidine. The usual dose is from 30 mg to 60 mg. It has been claimed that respiratory depression, nausea and vomiting are less than are usually associated with morphine and pethidine. Profound hypotension can occur after larger doses of dihydrocodeine and this, together with its relatively weak analgesic action, limits its usefulness in labour. Dihydrocodeine is exempt from the Misuse of Drugs Regulations, although addiction has been recorded.

5. Inhalational Analgesia

The three agents in current use as inhalational analgesics in labour are nitrous oxide, Trilene (trichloroethylene) and Penthrane (methoxyflurane). These agents will be considered separately.

The inhalational analgesic techniques used by midwives can give a useful measure of pain relief to many women. Analgesia is usually not complete and a few women appear to obtain almost no relief. To extract the greatest possible benefit from relatively low, but inherently safe, concentrations of inhalational analgesics it is essential to understand and abide by correct methods of administration.

Nitrous oxide

The older methods of nitrous oxide analgesia have at last been abandoned with the withdrawal of the C. M. B.'s approval of nitrous oxide and air mixtures in 1970. The Minnitt's and allied machines may no longer be used by midwives and the only apparatus currently approved for midwives' use is the Entonox apparatus for the administration of nitrous oxide and oxygen.

Nitrous oxide and air mixtures have been abolished, not because they were ineffective but because they inevitably caused maternal and fetal hypoxia (oxygen lack). The Minnitt, Talley, Amwell and Jecta apparatus delivered a 50:50 nitrous oxide and air mixture. Because air contains 21 per cent of oxygen, the patient breathed only 10.5 per cent of oxygen and although this hypoxic mixture has been given to millions of women with apparent safety, the breathing of such a mixture must be regarded as a physiological trespass which is no longer justified with the availability of the Entonox apparatus. Moreover the Minnitt's and similar machines were often wildly inaccurate and sometimes delivered as little as 2 or 3 per cent of oxygen. While paying tribute to the work of Minnitt and Elam of Liverpool in pioneering nitrous oxide and air analgesia and admitting the benefits bestowed on countless women since 1933, the relegation of 'gas and air' machines to the obstetric museum is welcomed.

Non-hypoxic nitrous oxide and oxygen mixtures are now widely used for analgesia in the first and second stages of labour. The Lucy Baldwin apparatus is used in some hospitals but only the Entonox apparatus is approved for use by midwives on their own responsibility and subject to the following regulations which relate to any form of inhalational analgesia.

Central Midwives Boards' Regulations for Use of Inhalational Analgesia by Midwives. There is the general proviso that a midwife must not, on her own responsibility, use any analgesic method 'unless in the course of her training, whether before or after enrolment she has been thoroughly instructed in its use and is familiar with its dosage and methods of administration.' The following rules, introduced in 1955, apply specifically to inhalational analgesia administered by the unsupervised midwife.

A practising midwife must not on her own responsibility administer an inhalational analgesic unless:

1. She has, either before or after enrolment, received at an institution approved by the Board for the purpose, special instruction in the essentials of obstetric analgesia and has satisfied the institution or the Board that she is thoroughly proficient in the use of the apparatus.

2. The patient has at some time during the pregnancy been examined by a registered medical practitioner who has signed a certificate that he finds no contraindication to the administration of analgesia by a midwife and if any illness which required medical attention subsequently developed during the pregnancy, the midwife obtained confirmation from a medical practitioner that the certificate remained valid (C. M. B. England, 1955). The ruling in Scotland is that the patient has 'within one month before her confinement been examined by a registered medical practitioner' and certified fit for inhalational analgesia.

3. The ruling which required the presence of an acceptable third person during the administration has now been abolished.

The Entonox apparatus and premixed gases

The Entonox apparatus consists of two main parts. There is a cylinder of premixed nitrous oxide and oxygen gases in equal proportions and attached to the cylinder there is a combined reducing valve (pressure regulator) and demand valve.

Premixed gases

A cylinder of premixed gases contains an even mixture of 50 per cent of nitrous oxide and 50 per cent of oxygen. Both substances are in the gaseous state. The mixture remains remarkably constant in use. There is one vitally important exception to this statement. If the cylinder is exposed to a temperature of minus 7°C (19°F) or lower then separation of the two gases will occur. The heavier nitrous oxide will fall to the lower part of the cylinder. When the cylinder is turned on the emerging gas mixture will be composed almost entirely of oxygen from the upper part of the cylinder. Later, when almost all of the oxygen has been discharged the emerging gas will be almost pure nitrous oxide. The possibility of causing asphyxia by administering almost 100 per cent nitrous oxide will be apparent. If the cooled cylinder is in the horizontal position, the risk of delivering a severely hypoxic mixture is less because the emerging mixture, although uneven, is more likely to contain both nitrous oxide and oxygen. This point is illustrated in Fig 2.

Air temperatures of minus 7°C and below do occur in Great Britain and occur frequently in other countries. There is no simple, certain method of detecting that separation of the gases has occurred. The presence of ice or condensation on the cylinder should arouse suspicion but the absence of these signs does not guarantee safety. The only absolute safeguard is to ensure that cylinders of premixed gases are never exposed to low temperatures.

Separation of the gases and the delivery of a profoundly hypoxic mixture is the only potential danger of an otherwise most useful and safe apparatus.

Premixed gas cylinders are available in 500 litre, 2000 litre and 5000 litre sizes. The 500 litre sizes are easily portable and are intended for domiciliary use. The larger sizes are for hospital use. The 2000 litre size is transportable on a trolley. The 5000

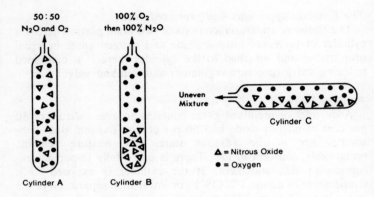

Fig. 2 The effect of cooling and position on premixed gases in cylinders. Cylinder A is a normal, uncooled cylinder and delivers a 50:50 mixture in any position. Cylinder B is a cooled vertical cylinder. The nitrous oxide is at the bottom. This cylinder will first deliver almost pure oxygen and later nearly pure nitrous oxide. Cylinder C is a cooled horizontal cylinder. Separation is less complete than in cylinder B because there is some mixing in the middle layer. An uneven, but probably less hypoxic mixture is delivered.

litre size may be connected to a pipeline supply to the labour ward.

A sub-committee of the Medical Research Council Committee on Nitrous oxide/oxygen Analgesia in Midwifery has made important recommendations on the safe handling and storage of premixed nitrous oxide and oxygen cylinders. The observance of these regulations should ensure safety and the regulations should be clearly understood by all who deal with these cylinders.

The M. R. C. sub-committee's recommendations are as follows:

500 litre cylinders for domiciliary use. (1). If a cylinder of premixed oxygen and nitrous oxide has been exposed to cold, the two gases may separate. This may result in the patients receiving either an oxygen-deficient or a nitrous oxide-deficient mixture.

Observation of the following procedure will ensure safety at any time of the year. The gases may be remixed by warming the cylinder to a safe temperature and then agitating the contents by inverting the cylinder three times. A safe temperature is achieved either by keeping the cylinder in the delivery room or in a room above 10°C for at least two hours before use, or by placing it in warm water, at body temperature, for five minutes. Hot water must not be used for this purpose and care should be taken not to allow water into the valve. (2). The following warning label should be indelibly attached to all 500 litre cylinders 'Do not store in the open. Always protect from cold. Immediately before use ensure that the cylinder has been adequately warmed and then invert it completely three times. Never use grease or oil on the valve.'

Because it is impractical to invert the large cylinders by hand the following recommendations are made. The responsibility for implementing these recommendations rests with the hospital authority and the sub-committee of the M. R. C. states that midwives and medical staff cannot be held responsible for separation of gas in 2000 litre and 5000 litre cylinders.

2000 litre and 5000 litre cylinders. (1). On receipt, the cylinders should be date-marked and before use stored in a horizontal position for 24 hours in an area maintained at a temperature above 10°C (50°F) but not exceeding 45°C (113°F).

(2). During delivery from the storage area to the final destination point in the hospital the cylinder must not be exposed to a freezing temperature for more than 10 minutes.

It should be noted that midwives using 500 litre cylinders in domiciliary practice are responsible for the proper handling of these cylinders and that the hospital authority is responsible for the larger cylinders. Responsibility is not placed upon the manufacturer. Cylinders may be cooled during transport to the hospital and this is the reason for advising storage at 10°C or higher for 24 hours. It has been suggested that excessive cooling of the master cylinder of a hospital piped Entonox system might result from the very high flow rates which may occur when multiple outlets are in use. This possibility has now been excluded by the fitting of a device which restricts flows to 300 litres/minute.

Cylinder Requirements: The average volume of premixed gases used in a domiciliary confinement is about 500 litres, but requirements vary widely. It is recommended that two 500 litre cylinder be taken to each confinement. Three cylinders may be required for some primigravidae. Each cylinder weighs approximately 7 kg (16 lbs) so that the total weight is considerable.

The Entonox apparatus

The Entonox apparatus combines the following features in a compact fashion.

1. A small reducing valve (pressure regulator) which reduces the high cylinder pressure to a safe working pressure.

2. A demand valve which allows gas to flow only when the patient inhales from the face mask. The Entonox apparatus works on the 'demand' or 'intermittent flow' principle to economise on gases.

3. A small pressure (contents) gauge marked 0, $\frac{1}{4}$ and full. This gauge, unlike those on cylinders of nitrous oxide, indicates the amount of gas in the cylinder.

There is also a key with which to turn on the cylinder, a length of corrugated rubber tubing and a face mask. An expiratory valve next to the face mask ensures that, when the mask is properly applied to the face, each inspiration comes entirely from the cylinder and each expiration goes out into the atmosphere.

A non-interchangeable pin-index system allows the Entonox apparatus to be connected only to a cylinder of premixed 50:50 nitrous oxide and oxygen. These cylinders are identified by their having a blue colour with white bands or 'quarters' at the neck.

To prepare the Entonox apparatus for use: 1. Attach the Entonox to the cylinder of premixed gases by inserting the pins into the holes on the neck of the cylinder and tighten the retaining hand screw.

2. Turn on the cylinder with the key. There should be a brief hiss of gas which should cease at once.

3. Check the pressure (contents) gauge.

The apparatus is now ready for use.

After using the Entonox apparatus: 1. Turn off the cylinder with the key. Do not use great force.

2. Vent the apparatus by pressing the finger tips of both hands upwards on the under-surface of the Entonox. There will be a

brief hiss of gas. If the Entonox is not vented after use the demand valve may be damaged.

3. Wash the face mask in soapy water or cetavlon (Savlon). The face mask and rubber tubing may be sterilised by immersing in gluteraldehyde (Cidex) or chlorhexidine (Hibitane). The antiseptic must be carefully wahsed off before use. Rubber parts may also be boiled but repeated boiling causes deterioration. Deflate the rim of the mask before boiling. Pasteurisation in water at 70°C for 20 minutes is harmless and kills most bacteria including tubercle bacilli.

The properties of nitrous oxide

Nitrous oxide is a weak anaesthetic with a relatively strong analgesic action. When nitrous oxide is administered with 50 per cent of oxygen analgesia is satisfactory for many patients for normal labour and delivery, especially if pethidine has been given earlier in labour. Consciousness is not lost. A 50:50 mixture of nitrous oxide and oxygen is entirely free of harmful effects when given for not more than 12 hours and there are no absolute contraindications to the use of this mixture. Although consciousness is retained when the mixture is inhaled intermittently with contractions, if the mixture were inhaled continuously over many minutes then some patients would become unconscious. The margin between the analgesic concentration in the patient's blood and the concentration required to produce unconsciousness is quite small. Occasionally a patient will refuse inhalational analgesia because of her fear of the mask. Such a patient may find a plastic mouth-piece an acceptable substitute for a mask. Analgesic mixtures of nitrous oxide and oxygen do not cause significant respiratory depression, although nitrous oxide does cross the placental barrier. The high percentage of oxygen may be beneficial to the mother and the fetus. Uterine contractions are not inhibited. Mixtures of nitrous oxide and oxygen are not explosive but they do support combustion vigorously. Any explosion will, therefore, be more violent and flames will burn more brightly in an atmosphere of nitrous oxide and oxygen. The Entonox apparatus should be kept away from sources of ignition such as coal or gas fires. Entonox is almost odourless and rarely causes sickness.

The Technique of Nitrous Oxide and Oxygen Analgesia

Patients should be instructed in the technique of inhalational analgesia during pregnancy and the instructions should be briefly revised during labour. Most hospitals hold a class in inhalation analgesia for patients attending the antenatal clinic. Patients should be assured that they will not become unconscious and that they will gain substantial, although not necessarily complete relief from pain. The apparatus is demonstrated and the method of fitting the mask to the face is shown. The under surface of the mask is triangular in shape and the base of the triangle is fitted between the point of the chin and the lips while the narrow apex of the triangle fits over the bridge of the nose. Unless the mask is properly fitted then no gas will flow. Failure to apply the face mask properly is the commonest cause of failure to obtain analgesia. A common fault is to tilt the face mask so that one side is not in contact with the face. When gas flows a hissing noise is heard and this can be demonstrated to the patient. Some women are afraid of the mask and require reassurance that they will not suffocate and will be able to remove the mask at any time and that consciousness will not be lost. Such patients may accept a disposable tubular mouthpiece.

Nitrous oxide produces analgesia very rapidly and its effects wear off with equal rapidity when inhalation ceases. Analgesia comes on after inhaling nitrous oxide for about 20 seconds and is almost at its maximum after 45 to 60 seconds. Because nitrous oxide is taken up through the lungs, the rate and depth of respiration influence the rate of onset of analgesia. Fairly deep breathing at a normal rate is the most efficient type of respiration for inducing analgesia quickly. Very rapid and shallow breathing is inefficient. The first 150 ml of any inhalation are required to ventilate the dead space of the nose, mouth, pharynx, trachea and bronchi and nitrous oxide is not absorbed from this dead space. The percentage of a shallow breath reaching the alveoli and allowing gases to be transformed to the blood stream is relatively small. For example, if only 250 ml of gases are inhaled then only 100 ml are available for uptake. The rapid, panting type of breathing which some patients perform must be strongly discouraged.

Unless the midwife understands and applies the foregoing in-

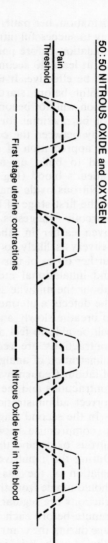

50:50 NITROUS OXIDE and OXYGEN

Pain Threshold

——— First stage uterine contractions

- - - Nitrous Oxide level in the blood

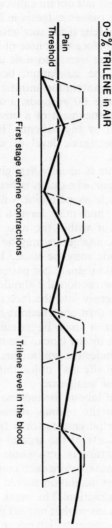

0·5% TRILENE in AIR

Pain Threshold

——— First stage uterine contractions

——— Trilene level in the blood

Fig. 3 The analgesic effects of nitrous oxide and Trilene.
The effect of nitrous oxide develops rapidly and wears off with equal rapidity.
The effect of Trilene develops more slowly but is sustained after a few contractions.

formation, her patient will not obtain satisfactory analgesia. The key to successful nitrous oxide analgesia in labour is to begin the inhalation before pain is felt. If the analgesic mixture is inhaled for at least 20 seconds before the onset of pain, then analgesia will be effective. It is quite wrong to wait until a contraction is painful before starting the inhalation, because the analgesic action will not become apparent for another 20 seconds and will not be maximal for some 60 seconds. Fortunately there is a delay between the commencement of a uterine contraction and the appreciation of pain by the patient. This time lag must be used to build up an analgesic level of nitrous oxide in the patient's blood (Fig. 3).

Nitrous oxide analgesia is usually first given towards the end of the first stage of labour when pain is becoming more severe. Narcotic analgesics, such as pethidine will usually have been given earlier in labour and may have a persisting effect. If delivery is likely to occur within the next two or three hours, further doses of narcotic analgesics may be harmful to the fetus and inhalational methods may be used. In the first stage of labour the midwife should palpate her patient's abdomen. When she detects a uterine contraction she should instruct her patient to breathe slowly and deeply into the face mask. Some patients will be able to feel their own contractions before pain is felt. If contractions are regular it may be possible to time the administration of analgesia by the clock. The modern management of labour frequently includes the continuous recording of uterine contractions and the midwife may utilise this information for the correct administration of analgesia.

In the second stage of labour the technique must be modified to compromise between the optimal method of administering nitrous oxide and the requirements for a spontaneous delivery. During the expulsive efforts of the second stage the regular inhalation of the gas mixture is impossible and so the patient should inhale from the mask before each contraction. When contractions are regular then inhalation should be commenced one minute before each contraction. The mask may be held on the face during the contractions so that nitrous oxide and oxygen are inhaled at the brief inspirations which occur between the sustained expulsive efforts. During crowning of the head the patient should inhale continuously from the mask. This will discourage unwanted expulsive efforts and increase the level of analgesia. Although self-administration is usual, it is sometimes more satisfactory for the midwife to hold the mask correctly on the patient's face. This is likely to be helpful if the patient is agitated or poorly instructed. Should the cylinder become empty the conscious patient will at once experience the greatest difficulty in breathing and would pull the mask from her face. Sometimes a patient will reject the mask at delivery and she should be allowed to do so.

The Entonox apparatus may also be used during delivery of the placenta and during vaginal examinations in labour. Breathing regularly from the face mask may prevent premature expulsive efforts during the first stage of labour. Inhalational analgesia may be used during breech delivery and during forceps delivery to augment pudendal nerve block. The Entonox apparatus will not provide adequate analgesia by itself for forceps delivery. Analgesia is not really adequate for the performance of an episiotomy and for this procedure the midwife should first infiltrate the perineum with local anaesthetic solution.

General Comments

Gases in cylinders are virtually dry, whereas the normal room air contains a considerable quantity of water. Every exhalation is saturated with water vapour and the prolonged inhalation of dry gases accentuates the water loss which always occurs to some extent during labour. Hyperventilation will further increase water loss through the lungs. Hyperventilation, if extreme, may lower the maternal blood carbon dioxide tension to levels which impair placental circulation and cause fetal hypoxia. The tendency of some patients to hyperventilate when breathing from a face mask must be corrected. Maternal tetany may follow hyperventilation. These complications are rare and will not occur with proper technique. There is evidence which supports the view that the inhalation of a 50:50 mixture of nitrous oxide and oxygen in the second stage can improve fetal oxygenation and reduce metabolic acidosis in cases of fetal distress.

About 50 per cent of women in normal labour will obtain good, although rarely complete pain relief from a pethidine, nitrous oxide and oxygen sequence of analgesia. A few apparently normal women seem to get very little pain relief from a 50:50 mixture of nitrous oxide and oxygen. Other women may become confused and unco-operative but this is uncommon with 50 per cent of nitrous oxide. The sub-committee of the Medical Research Council felt that there was a need for concentrations of nitrous oxide greater than 50 per cent in certain abnormal types of labour and delivery. Mixtures of up to 70 per cent nitrous oxide in oxygen may conveniently be got from the Lucy Baldwin apparatus which midwives may use only under medical supervision. This apparatus is described below.

Properly administered nitrous oxide and oxygen mixtures will often give a reasonable degree of analgesia. If pain relief is not satisfactory the explanation may be found in some fault in the apparatus, the technique of administration or there may be an obsetric abnormality causing unusually painful labour. Even properly administered nitrous oxide may fail to relieve pain. In the Medical Research Council study 30 per cent of patients were helped only slightly or not at all.

Common Causes of Apparent Failure of Analgesia with Nitrous Oxide

1. The cylinder is empty. Check pressure (contents) gauge.

2. The face mask is not being fitted closely to the face and no gases are being delivered. A common fault. The Entonox and Lucy Baldwin apparatus emit a hissing sound with each inspiration when gases are being delivered to the patient.

3. The administration is faulty. Inhalation must be commenced before the pain. Administration may have been started too late in labour.

4. The patient is unco-operative, uninstructed or psychologically unsuited to inhalational analgesia.

5. Labour is abnormally painful. Think of occipito-posterior positions, inco-ordinate uterine action and cephalopelvic disproportion.

6. The patient is one of approximately 30 per cent who do not obtain pain relief from 50 per cent nitrous oxide.

The Lucy Baldwin Apparatus. The Lucy Baldwin apparatus is a modified dental anaesthetic machine and is not approved by the C. M. B. for use by midwives on their own responsibility. Variable percentages of nitrous oxide and oxygen are obtainable. According to the dial setting any percentage of nitrous oxide between 50 and 70 per cent can be delivered. By unlocking a lock on the apparatus an 80 per cent concentration of nitrous oxide in oxygen can be delivered. This mixture can produce anaesthesia and should never be used by a midwife. Pure oxygen can be delivered if required.

For normal labour a 50:50 mixture of nitrous oxide and oxygen will usually be satisfactory. The main advantage of the Lucy Baldwin apparatus is that a 70:30 nitrous oxide and oxygen ratio is available for more painful labours. When 70 per cent of nitrous oxide is used the risk of the patient becoming drowsy or confused is increased.

In the Lucy Baldwin apparatus the nitrous oxide and oxygen are not premixed but are obtained from separate cylinders (two for each gas). Only one cylinder of each gas should be turned on. The remaining cylinder of each gas should be full. When the cylinder in use becomes empty the full cylinder is turned on and the empty cylinder is replaced by a full cylinder. The pressure gauges on the oxygen cylinders indicate the contents of the cylinders. The pressure gauges on the nitrous oxide cylinders do not indicate the state of fullness of the cylinders. Nitrous oxide pressure gauges indicate essentially the same pressure whether the cylinder is full or almost empty. The Lucy Baldwin apparatus is well suited to use with piped gases rather than cylinders.

A safety device is incorporated which permits the patient to breathe only room air if the supply of either gas should fail. The Lucy Baldwin apparatus is acceptably accurate in all likely conditions of use. If the gas flows are very low, the oxygen percentage falls but these very low flows are unlikely to occur with patients in labour who usually breathe vigorously. Like all other inhalational analgesic apparatus for use in labour, the Lucy Baldwin apparatus delivers no analgesic gases unless the patient inhales from a properly fitted face mask.

Trilene (trichlorothylene)

Trilene is the proprietary brand of trichloroethylene in use in the United Kingdom and the name Trilene will be used because it is the one by which this agent is best known.

The properties of Trilene

Trilene is a liquid which is coloured blue by the addition of a dye in order to distinguish it from other liquid anaesthetics. Trilene has a high boiling point for an anaesthetic agent (87°C) and a low volatility. Trilene evaporates slowly and so only low concentrations of Trilene vapour are attainable for inhalation by the patient. It is, therefore, difficult to produce deep anaesthesia with Trilene, but it is relatively easy to obtain lower, analgesic concentrations of Trilene vapour without the risk of producing anaesthesia.

Trilene can be decomposed by light and heat to form toxic substances such as phosgene. Trilene must, therefore, be stored in dark glass bottles or metal containers and kept away from heat. It has been suggested that the heat of a cigarette may decompose the Trilene vapour in a patient's breath and smoking should be avoided for some hours after Trilene analgesia.

Trilene, in the concentrations used for analgesia is not explosive when mixed with air and so can be safely used in the presence of a source of ignition such as a fire. Decomposition of Trilene may occur if there is a fire in the room.

Trilene can react with hot soda lime to form substances capable of producing cranial nerve palsies and encephalitis. Soda lime is, of course, not used in Trilene inhalers. The potential danger is that a patient who has inhaled Trilene vapour during labour may exhale this vapour into an anaesthetic circuit incorporating soda lime, should a general anaesthetic be given for delivery. The midwife should inform the anaesthetist that Trilene has been administered during labour.

Anaesthetic concentrations of Trilene sometimes cause cardiac arrhythmias but serious arrhythmias have not been reported with the analgesic concentrations approved for midwives' use (0.35 per cent and 0.5 per cent Trilene in air). If adrenaline is injected during Trilene anaesthesia the risk of cardiac arrhythmias and even cardiac arrest is increased. Although cardiac arrest has not occurred following the injection of adrenaline during the use of a C. M. B. approved Trilene inhaler, the remote possibility exists, at least in theory. It therefore seems prudent to avoid the use of adrenaline during Trilene analgesia and if local anaesthetic solutions are used for perineal infiltration or pudendal nerve block they should preferably not contain adrenaline when Trilene is being inhaled.

The concentrations of Trilene vapour used in midwifery have themselves negligible depressant effect on maternal and neonatal respiration. Where, as is often the case, narcotic analgesics have also been administered the combined depressant action of the two types of analgesics may occasionally become significant. Trilene, like all anaesthetic and analgesic agents, crosses the placental barrier and it is generally and probably correctly believed that Trilene sometimes causes the infant to be rather inactive and sleepy at birth. This effect is most likely to be observed when pethidine or other narcotic analgesics have also been given during labour. It is not suggested that Trilene analgesia seriously depresses normal infants.

The inhalation of Trilene vapour occasionally causes the mother's breathing to become very rapid (tachypnoea). The respirations are then also usually very shallow. This is an inefficient type of respiration which may cause maternal hypoxia. Respiratory rates of up to 100 per minute have been recorded. This effect of Trilene must be distinguished from the voluntary hyperventilation which some patients perform. Tachypnoea is an indication for stopping the inhalation of Trilene.

Pure Trilene does not damage the liver. The basis for the belief that it does so is that workers who are constantly exposed to impure industrial trichloroethylene may suffer liver damage. Trilene does not damage the kidneys.

It must be stressed that the foregoing effects of Trilene are very rare and are nearly all preventable. They should not be regarded as objections to the informed used of Trilene in the accurately controlled concentrations obtainable from the inhalers approved by the C. M. B. (Tecota Mark 6 and Emotril Automatic). Serious side-effects are more likely to occur when higher and uncontrolled concentrations of Trilene vapour are inhaled. Midwives are warned against the use of unapproved inhalers. A number of deaths have occurred with certain Trilene inhalers which are sometimes used by general practitioners and obstetricians and which are still found in some hospitals. These unapproved inhalers may deliver very high concentrations of Trilene vapour.

Commoner side effects of Trilene analgesia are nausea and vomiting. Drowsiness and lack of co-operation may occur. If any of these effects appear then the concentration of Trilene should be reduced to 0.35 per cent or the inhalation should be discontinued.

Trilene has rather a sweet smell which some patients find unpleasant, while others may believe that they are getting a 'stronger' analgesic because of the smell. The smell is usually no longer noticed after a few breaths.

Trilene does not inhibit uterine contractions in the concentrations used by midwives. There is no reduction in the inspired oxygen percentage and Trilene and air does not cause hypoxia. There is of course normally no increase in the percentage of oxygen inhaled. It is possible to increase the percentage of oxygen inhaled by running a supply of oxygen alongside the inspiratory port of the Trilene inhaler. A hood has been designed to fit over the top of the Emotril (and Cardiff) inhaler. Oxygen is run into the hood and the patient receives an oxygen-rich mixture. From one to five litres/minute may be used and the patient receives up to 50 per cent of oxygen at the higher flow rates.

Trilene and air was associated with progressive fetal hypoxia and acidosis in the presence of fetal distress. These deliveries were conducted in the dorsal position and this position has been subsequently shown to cause fetal acidosis unless modified by elevation of the right buttock in order to relieve compression of the inferior vena cava. Nevertheless Trilene and air was associated with greater hypoxia than was Entonox and there is a case to be made out for administering extra oxygen in the presence of fetal distress.

Trilene is undoubtedly an effective analgesic agent and in this respect it is at least as effective as 50 per cent nitrous oxide and is perhaps marginally better. When properly administered from one of the C. M. B. approved inhalers, Trilene analgesia is safe. Because of the potential dangers of higher and uncontrolled concentrations of Trilene, the C. M. B. have introduced strict regulations governing the use of Trilene by midwives.

Central midwives boards' regulations. The regulations

relating to the use of any inhalational analgesic are applicable and are listed on page 57. Midwives who have already been fully instructed in nitrous oxide analgesia are considered to be capable of administering Trilene on their own responsibility when they have attended a demonstration on the use of the apparatus (C. M. B. England). The Scottish Board requires such midwives to attend one lecture on Trilene and to administer it to three patients.

There are rigid specifications relating to the accuracy of Trilene inhalers for midwives' use. The two principal factors which affect the concentration of Trilene vapour delivered by an inhaler are the temperature of the liquid and the depth of the patient's respirations. With the simpler, unapproved types of inhaler the percentage of Trilene vapour delivered will increase to potentially dangerous levels in a warm room and decrease in a cold room. The approved inhalers compensate automatically for changes in temperature and the Trilene vapour concentration is not greatly affected by variations in the depth of respiration.

Only two Trilene inhalers comply with the C. M. B.'s specifications. These inhalers are the Tecota Mark 6 and the Emotril (Automatic) trichloroethylene analgesia inhalers.

The Tecota Mark 6 and Emotril (automatic) inhalers. Although externally these two Trilene inhalers do not look alike they both comply with the specifications of the C. M. B. (TECOTA is derived from TEmperature COmpensated Trilene Air. EMOTRIL is derived from the names of its inventors, Epstein and Macintosh of Oxford). They can deliver either 0.5 per cent or 0.35 per cent of Trilene vapour in air. The oxygen content of the inhaled mixture is therefore essentially that of room air (21 per cent). These inhalers are very accurate when the room temperature lies between the specified range of from 13°C (55°F) to 35°C (95°F). This is because the effects of variations in temperature are automatically compensated for, within this range of temperatures. The effects of different respiratory volumes are also compensated for. The inhalers are robust, will operate in any position and the contents are unspillable.

The C. M. B.'s regulations require that the accuracy of these inhalers be assessed yearly to comply with the specifications of the British Standards Institution (formerly of the National Physical Laboratory). When the test has been satisfactorily completed a seal is applied. This seal is inscribed with the letters B. S. T. and the month and the year in which the test was performed. For example, if the test was performed in October, 1977, the symbols B. S. T., 10, 77 would be used. The inhalers are returned to the makers for annual testing. It is the midwife user's responsibility to arrange for this testing, which usually involves loss of use of the inhaler for up to a month.

The Tecota Mark 6 and Emotril inhalers work on the draw-over principle. When the patient inhales from a properly fitting face mask her inspiratory effort draws room air into the inhaler. A proportion of this air is then drawn into the vaporising chamber which contains liquid Trilene. Trilene vapour is then mixed with this air. To increase the surface area of Trilene available for vaporisation a number of wicks, similar to those used in paraffin lamps, dip into the liquid Trilene and are soaked in the liquid.

Some of the air drawn into the inhaler by-passes the vaporising chamber and goes directly to the patient. The proportion of air going to the vaporising chamber is automatically increased when the room temperature falls and is decreased when the temperature rises. Thus the final percentage of Trilene vapour reaching the patient is constant despite variations in temperature, at least within the specified range 13°C to 35°C.

There are two settings on the inhalers so that a minimum or weak mixture of 0.35 per cent of Trilene vapour in air and a maximum or normal mixture of 0.5 per cent of Trilene vapour in air are obtainable. Each inhaler has a filling orifice and a small window to permit inspection of the level of liquid Trilene. Only the Emotril (Automatic) inhaler has a circular dial on its upper surface. This dial has on it the words 'Operating Field' and 'Out of Action'. The dial indicates whether the room temperature lies within the range 13°C and 35°C and is in fact a thermometer. When the temperature is within the prescribed range the needle will lie within the section inscribed 'Operating Field'. It is understood that the manufacture of the Emotril inhaler has now ceased. Its use by midwives continues to be authorised.

It is essential to realise that, just as with the Entonox and

Lucy Baldwin apparatus, the patient will receive no analgesia from a Trilene inhaler unless she inhales from a properly fitting face mask.

The technique of Trilene analgesia

The indications for Trilene and air analgesia and the method of administration are essentially the same as those already described for nitrous oxide and oxygen. Inhalations are given with the contractions in the first stage of labour, before the contractions in the second stage, and continously during crowning of the head. Breathing should be fairly deep and quite slow. Rapid, shallow breathing is to be avoided and rarely this type of breathing may be caused by Trilene and is then not under the patient's control.

Trilene possesses one important property which nitrous oxide lacks. The elimination of Trilene from the blood and tissues is very slow and so Trilene progressively accumulates in the body with each period of inhalation. In contrast to nitrous oxide, Trilene is not excreted almost immediately by the lungs when inhalation ceases. The complete elimination of Trilene from the body may take many hours. Consequently when Trilene vapour has been administered with a few contractions, a background level of analgesia will have built up and will persist between contractions. This cumulative property of Trilene forms the basis for the not strictly accurate, but often repeated statement that Trilene is a very rapidly acting analgesic agent. The apparent rapidity of action is explained by the existence of analgesic levels of Trilene in the blood at the time of onset of a contraction. This level can be easily topped up by further inhalations during the contraction. This state will not be achieved until Trilene has been administered during several contractions. When background analgesia has been attained, it then becomes less important to administer the Trilene vapour during the early, painless part of each uterine contraction in the first stage of labour. This may be an advantage of Trilene over nitrous oxide for those who cannot or will not expend the time and care necessary for the proper administration of nitrous oxide (Fig. 3, p. 53).

In a few patients the cumulative effects of Trilene prove to be disadvantageous. Drowsiness, disorientation and lack of co-operation with the midwife may occur. When these signs develop the concentration of Trilene vapour should be reduced from 0.5 per cent or the administration of Trilene vapour should be stopped. It has been recommended that Trilene should not be administered for longer than six hours. Such prolonged use would seldom if ever be contemplated today and a limit of one or two hours seems more realistic.

The midwife has the choice of administering either 0.5 per cent or 0.35 per cent of Trilene vapour in air. It is a sound principle of analgesic therapy to administer a relatively large and probably effective dose of an analgesic drug initially and to maintain analgesia with subsequent smaller doses. Therefore, an 0.5 per cent concentration of Trilene vapour should be used for most patients, especially if the administration is first begun in the painful, late first stage of labour. The lower concentration should be used if the patient becomes drowsy or unco-operative with the higher concentration. The lower concentration may also be preferred for those patients who have already received large doses of narcotic analgesics.

Indications for discontinuing or reducing the concentration of Trilene

Tachypnoea (very rapid and shallow respirations).
A slow or irregular pulse.
Drowsiness, disorientation or loss of co-operation.
Nausea and vomiting.
Strong objection by the patient to this form of analgesia.

If adrenaline is to be injected (perhaps combined with a local anaesthetic solution) it is probably wiser to discontinue the inhalation of Trilene. Nitrous oxide and oxygen may be safely used instead.

In the presence of fetal distress and placental insufficiency the higher concentration of oxygen obtained with the Entonox apparatus may make it preferable to Trilene and air inhalers. Alternatively an oxygen-enrichment device may be used.

Penthrane (methoxyflurane)

Penthrane is the trade name for methoxyflurane, an anaesthetic and analgesic agent introduced into clincal practice in 1959 and approved for use by unsupervised midwives by the C. M. B. in 1970 and by the C. M. B. for Scotland in 1972.

Penthrane is a colourless liquid with a not unpleasant sweetish odour.

The boiling point is very high for an anaesthetic agent (105°C) and the volatility is low. Penthrane is non-explosive and may be used in the presence of an open fire. Penthrane is not decomposed by exposure to light and does not decompose in contact with soda lime. Penthrane, or one of its breakdown products, appears to cause renal damage in a few patients after prolonged deep anaesthesia. There was no evidence of such effects in a series of obstetric patients who received 0.35 per cent Penthrane for analgesia.

The concentration of Penthrane vapour used for analgesia in midwifery (0.35 per cent) does not significantly depress maternal respiration and produces no cardiovascular side-effects. Tachypnoea is uncommon. Uterine contractions are unaffected in established labour. Penthrane crosses the placental barrier. The injection of weak solutions of adrenaline (1:200 000 or less) along with local anaesthetics is considered safe during Penthrane analgesia.

Penthrane has many similarities to Trilene. Both agents are powerful analgesics with a sustained action in low concentration. The induction of a state of analgesia with Penthrane requires that the vapour be inhaled over a few minutes. As the inhalation is continued or repeated the level of Penthrane in the blood and tissues rises until a persisting analgesic level is attained. Thereafter, just as with Trilene, it is only necessary to top up with a further inhalation of Penthrane during each contraction. The complete elimination of Penthrane from the body takes some hours and the analgesic action is prolonged.

The C. M. B.'s for England and for Scotland have approved the Cardiff inhaler for use by midwives who have been instructed in the technique of Penthrane analgesia. No other inhaler has been approved and it is not permissible to use Penthrane in a Trilene inhaler.

The Cardiff inhaler. The Cardiff inhaler is a draw-over inhaler which delivers 0.35 per cent of Penthrane vapour in air. The effects of variations in room temperature and the depth of respirations on the output of Penthrane vapour are compensated for automatically. The Cardiff inhaler is a development of the Tecota Mark 6 Trilene inhaler, to which it bears an obvious resemblance. The Cardiff inhaler is coloured bright green and there is no means of varying the vapour concentration. A safety feature, intended to prevent filling with the wrong liquid, is that the filling orifice has been modified so that only a Penthrane bottle can be attached. Perhaps it would be over-critical to point out that it would be possible to put other liquids into a Penthrane bottle. If the Cardiff inhaler is overheated it could deliver up to 0.5 per cent Penthrane. This might occur after storage in a hot cupboard or in a car on a hot day and in such circumstances the inhaler should be kept at normal room temperature for an hour before use.

Cardiff inhalers are tested before delivery by the British Standards Institution and a seal is appended. Inhalers must be retested every year. A seal bearing the month and year of testing is applied. The oxygen enrichment device described for use with the Tecota Mark 6 may be used with the Cardiff inhaler.

The technique of Penthrane analgesia

The technique and principles described for the administration of Trilene analgesia are applicable to Penthrane and need not be repeated here. With the Cardiff inhaler there is no weak and strong vapour available and 0.35 per cent must be used exclusively. A weaker setting has been considered unnecessary because Penthrane accumulates in the body to a lesser extent than Trilene. This concentration is equivalent to approximately 0.5 per cent of Trilene vapour. Because Penthrane vapour must be inhaled for about five minutes before a good analgesic effect is attained it has been suggested that the Cardiff inhaler should first be used continuously for three to five minutes and that thereafter the administration should proceed in the usual intermittent manner. This suggestion appears sound. Penthrane sometimes induces a feeling of detachment or indifference in the patient and characteristically she may lie peacefully with her eyes closed, although not asleep.

Entonox, Trilene or Penthrane?

Nitrous oxide and oxygen analgesia has some definite points

of difference from Trilene or Penthrane analgesia. The Entonox apparatus delivers 50 per cent of oxygen and this has theoretical advantages, particularly in cases of fetal distress, placental insufficiency, premature labour and pre-eclampsia. Trilene and Penthrane are administered with air which is adequate for most patients and cannot fairly be considered to be a disadvantage in the normal patient. Extra oxygen can be entrained.

The rapid uptake and elimination of nitrous oxide necessitate greater attention to the timing of inhalations in relation to the uterine contractions but are widely believed to avoid the drowsiness and lack of co-operation sometimes seen when Trilene and Penthrane have accumulated in the body. On the other hand, the analgesic effect of Trilene and Penthrane persists between the contractions and is present at the onset of each ensuing contraction.

If cost is a consideration, then Trilene is the cheapest agent. The cost of Penthrane and Entonox is roughly similar. In domiciliary practice the greater portability of the Trilene and Penthrane inhalers may be advantageous.

Extensive trials of the three agents were conducted in 1968 in various hospitals in South Wales by midwives and anaesthetists. The results are interesting and illustrate some of the difficulties involved in assessing analgesia in labour. The details will be found in the *British Medical Journal*, **3**, 259) and these articles are commended to anyone seriously interested in the subject.

In the first trials the anaesthetists gave Penthrane or nitrous oxide in varying concentrations according to the patients' requirements and sometimes continuously during the period of administration. In these rather artificial circumstances the anaesthetists and the midwives considered that Penthrane gave slightly better analgesia than nitrous oxide and oxygen. The more relevant trials were the field trials in which the midwives administered nitrous oxide and oxygen, Trilene and Penthrane in the standard concentrations used by midwives and by intermittent inhalations. In these field trials the midwives considered that Penthrane gave better pain relief than nitrous oxide or Trilene and that nitrous oxide was the least effective analgesic, but the differences were small. The patients were unable to distinguish significantly between the pain relieving action of the three agents. The midwives considered that more patients became unco-operative with Penthrane than with Trilene or nitrous oxide. Despite this adverse comment, the midwives preferred Penthrane over the two other agents. With each agent there were nearly 30 per cent of mothers who stated that their pain had been relieved only slightly or not at all. A recent national survey of obstetric analgesic methods has indicated that Penthrane is not extensively used outside the Cardiff area.

One would be justified in concluding that the differences between the analgesic efficiency of Penthrane, Trilene and nitrous oxide are small, if indeed they are significant at all in clinical practice. Perhaps Penthrane is the best analgesic by a small margin, but is more likely to cause loss of co-operation. Penthrane is said to be especially suitable for short but painful labours and for anxious patients. Setting aside the possible advantages of the increased oxygen content of pre-mixed gases, the choice of agent can usually be left to the midwife who may have preferences based on fortunate or unfortunate experiences with one or other drug and perhaps on the influence of her teachers and textbooks.

6. Local Anaesthetics and Regional Analgesia

A chapter on the local anaesthetic drugs and the commoner techniques of regional analgesia is included in this book, because midwives are now authorised to use local anaesthetics for in-filtration of the perineum and thereafter to perform episiotomy and because increasing use is now being made of regional analgesia for delivery and for pain relief in the first stage of labour. The C. M. B. has authorised the topping-up of epidural analgesia by suitably trained midwives and has required midwives to participate in advanced techniques of analgesia under medical supervision. This progressive attitude justifies a fairly detailed description of the technique of epidural analgesia. The C. M. B. for Scotland is presently considering the approval of the topping-up of epidural analgesia by midwives.

A knowledge of the doses and toxic effects of the local anaesthetic agents is, of course, a prerequisite to their safe use. An understanding of the various regional techniques and their effects on the mother, the fetus and on uterine action is necessary if the midwife is to care for her patient effectively in labour when these techniques are used. The terms regional analgesia and conduction analgesia mean essentially the same. They imply the production of insensibility to pain by the in-terruption of the conduction of sensory impulses from a part of the body by the injection of local anaesthetic into or alongside the nerve or nerves supplying the part. Examples of regional analgesia are pudendal nerve block, paracervical block and epidural analgesia. Many of these techniques can have far-reaching effects, some of which are beneficial and some of which are potentially harmful. The midwife will often be the first to detect and to initiate the treatment of the side-effects of regional analgesia.

It may be thought that the use of some of the more complex

methods of regional analgesia is yet another step away from normal midwifery. In fact this is not necessarily so when these techniques are used in the management of already existing abnormalities. For example, the use of continuous epidural analgesia in patients with inco-ordinate uterine action will often be followed by the development of a more normal type of uterine action as well as by complete relief of distressing pain. Because of this Caesarean section may sometimes be avoided in such patients. Every midwife has seen many patients who have not obtained adquate analgesia from the routine narcotic drugs and inhalational techniques and who would have benefitted from the use of regional analgesia.

Local anaesthetic agents

Although more correctly described as local analgesics, because following their injection pain is relieved but sensations such as touch and temperature appreciation are usually unaffected, the term local anaesthetic is in such common use that it will be employed. It is important that the patient and the midwife should understand that the ability to feel touch and to appreciate the temperature of lotions applied to the skin does not imply that analgesia is not present.

Mode of action of local anaesthetics

The precise mode of action of local anaesthetics is uncertain, but they are capable of blocking the conduction of impulses along nerves. This blocking effect can be achieved at the fine nerve endings in the tissues as in local infiltration of the perineum or the local anaesthetic may be injected into or alongside nerve trunks. The local anaesthetic may be injected into the cerebrospinal fluid so that the nerve roots and perhaps the spinal cord itself are affected. This is the technique of spinal (subarachnoid) analgesia which is seldom used in Great Britain, but is still widely used in many other countries.

In general the thinner nerve fibres which transmit the sensation of pain and which carry impulses in the autonomic nervous system are more easily blocked than the thicker fibres which transmit motor impulses to the muscles and carry the sensations of touch and temperature appreciation. Consequently nerve blocks are followed by analgesia within the area supplied by the nerve and there is usually also dilatation of blood vessels in that area due to the blockage of sympathetic nerve fibres. Muscular relaxation is usually present but this does not necessarily imply paralysis of the muscles. The relaxation of the abdominal muscles which occurs during epidural analgesia and is sufficient to permit the performance of Caesarean section is due mainly to interruption of the *sensory* side of the reflex arcs involved in the maintenance of muscle tone. It is still possible for the patient under epidural blockade to push *voluntarily* and to deliver her baby spontaneously, provided, of course, that there are no mechanical difficulties to be overcome.

Local anaesthetic drugs and adrenaline

The local anaesthetics in general use in the United Kingdom for regional analgesia and local infiltration are: lignocaine (Xyolcaine, Xylotox, lidocaine U. S. P.); prilocaine (Citanest, propitocaine U. S. P.); bupivacaine (Marcain).

Procaine (Novocaine) is now rarely used because it has a short duration of action and sometimes produces less intense analgesia in comparison with lignocaine and prilocaine. Lignocaine is to-day the standard local anaesthetic agent and is a safe and efficient drug, provided that the approved dose is not exceeded. Prilocaine is even safer than lignocaine for single injections and is just as effective. Prilocaine is less suitable for repeated injections because then the development of methaemoglobinaemia is inevitable. Bupivacaine is a powerful drug which gives a longer duration of analgesia than the other local anaesthetics and is particularly useful for epidural blocks in the first stage of labour.

Lignocaine and prilocaine are normally used in strengths of 0.5 per cent or 1 per cent. Higher concentrations of lignocaine (1.5 per cent or 2 per cent) are sometimes used for epidural analgesia. For local infiltration, for pudendal nerve block and for paracervical block the concentration of these drugs should never exceed 1 per cent.

Bupivacaine is used in 0.25 per cent or 0.5 per cent solutions. This drug is not used for local infiltration of the perineum or for pudendal nerve block. The weaker solution is suitable for paracervical block and the stronger solution is often used for epidural analgesia. Many anaesthetists mix equal parts of 0.25 per cent and 0.5 per cent bupivacaine to obtain 0.375 per cent solution for epidural analgesia. This solution, it is claimed, causes very little motor weakness while producing usually excellent analgesia. The 0.5 per cent solution gives a longer duration of epidural analgesia than either of the weaker solutions.

The effect of adding adrenaline to local anaesthetic solutions should be understood. Adrenaline is a vasoconstictor and reduces the blood flow through the site of injection. This has two important results. First, the duration of analgesia is prolonged because the local anaesthetic is more slowly removed from the tissues. Secondly, the likelihood of toxic reactions is reduced because, owing to the reduced rate of removal of the local anaesthetic from the tissues, the blood levels of anaesthetic in the general circulation are not so high. Consequently larger doses of local anaesthetic may be used with safety when combined with adrenaline. The occurrence of toxic reations depends on the level of local anaesthetic drug in the general circulation.

Table 3 shows the safe doses of the three common local anaesthetics. Note that the addition of adrenaline increases the safe dose.

Table 3. Safe Doses of Local Anaesthetics

Drug	Without Adrenaline	With 1:200,000 Adrenaline
Lignocaine	200 mg (20 ml of 1%)	500 mg (50 ml of 1%)
Prilocaine	400 mg (40 ml of 1%)	600 mg (60 ml of 1%)
Bupivacaine	125 mg (25 ml of 0.5%)	125 mg (25 ml of 0.5%)

Provided that these maximum doses are not exceeded, toxic reactions should be very rare. There is always, however, the possibility of injecting a 'safe' dose into a blood vessel and then a toxic reaction is very likely to result. The risk of this is greatest when the site of injection lies close to a major artery but is avoidable by careful aspiration of blood before making the injection. The uterine artery may be punctured during paracervical block and the pudendal artery lies close to the pudendal nerve. The risk of puncturing a major vessel during infiltration of the stretched perineum is negligible.

Adrenaline itself is a potentially dangerous substance. An

overdose of adrenaline may cause ventricular arrhythmias, palpitations, hypertension and distressing feelings of anxiety. It is therefore essential that the strength of adrenaline in the local anaesthetic solution should not exceed 1 part per 200 000 (written 1:200 000). If this rule is adhered to, and the safe volumes of the various local anaesthetic solutions given in Table 3 are also adhered to, then toxic reactions to both adrenaline and the local anaesthetic should not occur, provided that intravascular injection is avoided. Because adrenaline makes almost no difference to the duration of action or the toxicity of bupivacaine, when used for epidural analgesia, many anaesthetists omit adrenaline when using bupivacaine.

The injection of adrenaline by any route during *anaesthesia* with Trilene may cause serious cardiac arrhythmias and has occasionally caused death. This catastrophe has not been reported in connection with Trilene analgesia administered from an Emotril or a Tecota Mark 6 inhaler. Nevertheless it seems prudent not to use local anaesthetic solutions containing adrenaline when Trilene is being inhaled or has recently been inhaled. Adrenaline may be inactivated by autoclaving.

Placental transfer of local anaesthetics

The placental transfer of lignocaine and prilocaine is free and the concentration of these agents in the fetal blood is usually about 70 per cent of the maternal blood concentration during epidural analgesia. The transfer of bupivacaine is much less extensive than that of most other agents. The fetal blood concentration is usually 20 or 30 per cent of the maternal blood concentration and this, together with its longer action and good analgesic effect make bupivacaine the agent of choice for epidural analgesia. Mepivacaine (Carbocaine) is usually avoided in obstetrics (except for subarachnoid analgesia) because its placental transfer is unrestricted and the maternal and fetal blood concentrations are approximately equal.

Toxic effects of local anaesthetics

Toxic effects may occur when an overdose of local anaesthetic drug is injected into the correct anatomical situation or when a normal dose is injected into a blood vessel. The toxic effects of all local anaesthetics are essentially the same, although the dose required to produce these effects varies with each agent.

The most important signs of a toxic reaction are those of cerebral excitation. At first there may be fine muscular twitchings, particularly affecting the facial muscles. Generalised convulsions then develop and consciousness is lost. During this phase the airway may be obstructed, the tongue may be bitten and the patient may vomit and may then inhale her stomach contents. Hypoxia from any or all of these causes is almost inevitable.

If a gross overdose has been given, then a phase of depression of the vital centres of the brain stem may follow the convulsive phase. Respirations become inadequate and may cease altogether and blood pressure and cardiac output fall.

Death may be caused by respiratory and circulatory failure or by hypoxia and respiratory obstruction in the convulsive phase.

A toxic effect which is almost specific to prilocaine among the local anaesthetics, is the development of methaemoglobinaemia. This is likely to produce visible cyanosis when approximately 1000 mg (100 ml of 1 per cent solution) have been given. Prilocaine freely crosses the placenta and so it must be assumed that both mother and fetus have methaemoglobinaemia. Because methaemoglobin does not carry oxygen, some degree of maternal and fetal hypoxia must occur. The use of prilocaine for repeated injections in paracervical or epidural blocks is therefore not recommended, although this drug is perfectly safe for pudendal nerve block and for infiltration of the perineum. Methaemoglobinaemia can be rapidly reversed by an intravenous injection of methylene blue in a dose of 1 mg per kg body weight.

The treatment of toxic reactions to local anaesthetics. In the convulsive stage the initial treatment consists in preventing respiratory obstruction and in treating hypoxia. It is realised that this may be difficult to carry out in the patient who is having generalised convulsions. The chin should be supported and if this can be done without damage to the teeth, then a mouth gag or bite block may be inserted. It is important to suck out any vomitus or mucus from the upper air passages to prevent aspiration of foreign material into the lungs.

Oxygen, if available, should be given and a high flow rate (8*l/min*) should be used.

Anticonvulsant drugs may be administered by the doctor. A small dose of thiopentone (Pentothal) may be given intravenously. From 50 mg to 100 mg should stop the convulsions and should not produce respiratory or cardiovascular depression. Suxamethonium (Scoline) may be used by an anaesthetist. The drug treatment of convulsions should not be attempted by the midwife, who should confine her efforts to clearing the airways and administering oxygen. Unless a gross overdose has been given, convulsions should soon stop spontaneously and the outlook is favourable if serious hypoxia and pulmonary aspiration have been avoided. Medical aid should, of course, be summoned.

If a gross overdose has been given then artificial ventilation of the lungs and even external cardiac massage may be indicated.

Allergy and hypersensitivity to local anaesthetics

These are mentioned principally in order to dismiss them as likely explanations for untoward reactions to local anaesthetics. True allergy is very rare and may be seen in persons such as dentists and workers in the pharmaceutical industry who regularly handle these drugs. An allergic reaction is likely to be manifest by skin rashes, joint pains and bronchospasm.

The existence of an extreme hypersensitivity to local anaesthetics, so that sudden death may follow the injection of a small dose, is doubted by many authorities and if it exists, then it is extremely rare.

Allergy and hypersensitivity have often provided convenient but probably inaccurate explanations for reactions due in fact to an overdose or an intravascular injection of local anaesthetic.

The use of hyaluronidase

Hyaluronidase (Hyalase) is a spreading agent and its use has been advocated to encourage the spread of local anaesthetics. The addition of hyaluronidase to a local anaesthetic solution will not compensate for a misplaced injection and its use is not recommended.

Local infiltration of the perineum for episiotomy

The use of local anaesthetics for perineal infiltration and the performance of episiotomy is now authorised by the Central Midwives Boards and the Joint Nursing and Midwife Council for Northern Ireland. The following account is concerned solely with the minimal infiltration required for the making of a painless episiotomy during a spontaneous delivery when the presenting part of the fetus is already stretching the perineum. Before forceps delivery it is customary to perform a more extensive infiltration and it should be remembered that in this situation the perineum may not be distended and thinned out. Repair of the episiotomy is likely to require a further more extensive infiltration in due course. The following is a simple procedure and free of risk if the recommended drugs and doses are adhered to and intravascular injection is avoided. The injection is made from a moving needle into a temporarily almost avascular region and so intravascular injection is very unlikely.

Technique. When the perineum is definitely being distended by the presenting part of the fetus, the patient should be placed in the dorsal position with her knees bent and separated. Alternatively the lateral position may be used if the midwife prefers this. The midwife must scrub up and wear sterile gloves and preferably also a sterile gown. The perineum is swabbed with an antispetic solution such as 0.5 per cent chlorhexidine (Hibitane) and the area draped with sterile towels.

A sterile 10 ml or 20 ml syringe is filled with sterile local anaesthetic solution. An 0.5 per cent solution of lignocaine (Xylocaine) or an 0.5 per cent solution of prilocaine (Citanest) is suitable. The C. M. B. stated (1967) that 10 ml of 0.5 per cent or 5 ml of 1 per cent solution of lignocaine or similar agent should be sufficient. In view of this, the use of 10 ml of an 0.5 per cent solution is recommended. The addition of adrenaline is not necessary for this simple infiltration of a small volume of solution. Note that the usual rubber-capped bottle is unsterile on the outside, although its contents are sterile and take care not to contaminate the fingers while drawing up the solution. The needle used for filling the syringe should be discarded and any unused solution should also be thrown out. A 22 S.W. G. needle at least 7.5 cm long is now attached to the syringe. When the perineum is somewhat relaxed between contractions the needle is inserted through the skin at the fourchette and slowly advanced in the line of the proposed episiotomy for 3 to 4 cm. After aspiration for blood, the needle is slowly withdrawn while 3 ml of solution are injected (Fig. 4). This injection is repeated on either side of the first injection so that a total of 9 to 10 ml of solution is used. A fan shaped area will now have been infiltrated. If two fingers of the other hand are inserted into the vagina during the injections, then accidental injection of the fetus is avoided. These injections should give adequate analgesia for the performance of an episiotomy within one or two minutes. It is important to allow this period of time for the production of good analgesia.

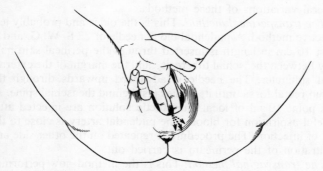

Fig. 4 Lines of injection of local anaesthetic solution for medio-lateral episiotomy.

Complications. In practice complications are most unlikely. Toxic reactions should not occur. Infection is avoided by proper aseptic and antiseptic technique. Injection of the fetus has occurred. If adrenaline is not used the remote possibility of avascular necrosis is avoided and the concomitant use of a trichloroethylene (Trilene) inhaler is completely safe.

The method of performing the following regional analgesic techniques will be described only in outline because they are not procedures which the midwife is authorised to perform. All of these techniques are at present in use in some British maternity hospitals and the midwife should be aware of the effects of those procedures on her patient.

Pudendal nerve block

A successful block of both pudendal nerves abolishes pain sensation in most of the perineum, vulva and vagina and relaxes the muscles of the pelvic floor. The uterus is not anaesthetised and therefore the pain of uterine contractions is not relieved. Pudendal nerve block is usually accompanied by infiltration of the perineum with local anaesthetic solution and is the most widely used method of analgesia for forceps delivery. Pudendal nerve block is not normally performed by midwives.

There are two basic methods of pudendal nerve block and several variations of these methods.

The transperineal method. This is the older and probably less effective method. A pudendal block needle of 22 S. W. G. and at least 10 cm in length is inserted through the perineal skin half-way between the ischial tuberosity and the margin of the external anal sphincter. The needle is advanced upwards through the ischio-rectal fossa until its tip lies just behind the ischial spine. At this point 10 ml of local anaesthetic solution are injected after careful aspiration for blood. The pudendal artery is close to the site of injection. The procedure is repeated on the other side and infiltration of the perineum is carried out.

The transvaginal method. This is the method now performed by many obstetricians and is more likely to be successful. The pudendal block needle is guarded by the second and third fingers and introduced into the vagina. The tip of the needle penetrates the vaginal wall at the level of the ischial spine and is placed just behind the ischial spine where 10 ml of local anaesthetic solution are injected. The opposite pudendal nerve is now blocked and the perineum is infiltrated. Some obstetricians use a guarded needle such as the Iowa trumpet for this procedure.

Bilateral pudendal nerve blocks and infiltration of the perineum involve the use of up to 40 ml of local anaesthetic solution. A 1 per cent solution of prilocaine (Citanest) is therefore suitable and the addition of adrenaline to the prilocaine is not essential. A 1 per cent solution of lignocaine (Xylocaine)

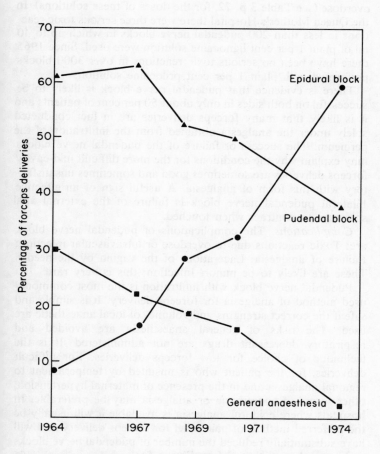

Fig. 5 The use of general anaesthesia, pudendal and epidural blocks for forceps deliveries in the Queen Mother's Hospital between 1964 and 1974. (Moir, D. D. (1976) in *Obstetric Anaesthesia and Analgesia*. London: Ballière Tindall.)

with 1:200 000 adrenaline is also satisfactory. The use of 40 ml of plain 1 per cent lignocaine involves the administration of an overdose (see Table 3 p. 72, for the doses of these solutions). In the Queen Mother's Hospital there were three serious toxic reactions in less than 200 pudendal nerve blocks in which up to 40 ml of plain 1 per cent lignocaine solution were used. Since 1965 there have been no serious toxic reactions in over 3000 blocks performed with plain 1 per cent prilocaine solution.

There is evidence that pudendal nerve block is likely to be successful on both sides in only about 50 per cent of patients and it is likely that many forceps deliveries are in fact conducted solely under the analgesia obtained from the infiltration of the perineum. The success or failure of the pudendal nerve blocks may explain why the conditions for the more difficult mid-cavity forceps deliveries are sometimes good and sometimes unsatisfactory with this form of analgesia. A useful sign of an effective bilateral pudendal nerve block is failure of the external anal sphincter to contract when touched.

Complications. The complications of pudendal nerve block are: Toxic reactions due to overdose or intravascular injection; Failure of analgesia; Lacerations of the vagina by the needle. These are likely to be minor. Infection; this is very rare.

Pudendal nerve block with infiltration is the most commonly used method of analgesia for forceps delivery. It is simple and safe if the correct strengths and volumes of local anaesthetic are used. The risks of general anaesthesia are avoided and respiratory depressant drugs are not administered. It is the technique of choice for low forceps deliveries. For difficult deliveries, for the patient who is unsuited by temperament to regional analgesia and in the presence of maternal hypertension, other forms of anaesthesia or analgesia may be preferable. In hospitals where epidural analgesia is available it will usually be the preferred method of pain relief for forceps delivery and will have substantially reduced the number of pudendal nerve blocks and general anaesthetics (see Figure 5).

Paracervical block

This form of regional analgesia can only be used in the first stage of labour. Paracervical block has been widely used in the

U. S. A. and in Scandinavia and has been used in many British hospitals. Paracervical block is sometimes referred to as uterosacral block because the injections are made alongside the cervix near the base of the uterosacral ligaments. The high incidence of fetal bradycardia associated with this otherwise useful technique has caused it to be abandoned in most centres.

The injections are usually made when the cervix is 5 cm to 7 cm (3 to 4 fingers) dilated and uterine contractions are well established and painful. The injections are difficult or even impossible when the cervix is nearly fully dilated or the presenting part is low in the pelvis. The aim is to block the paracervical ganglion or plexus (Frankenhauser's plexus) which contains all the nerves from the uterus.

The whole uterus is insensitive to pain after bilateral paracervical block and the pains of the first stage of labour are relieved or reduced in intensity. The success rate should be between 80 and 90 per cent. The lower birth canal is unaffected so that for forceps delivery additional analgesia will be required and for this purpose pudendal nerve block is usually chosen when a paracervical block has been used in the first stage of labour.

Technique. The technique is simple and the only equipment required is a sterile 20 ml syringe, a suitable local anaesthetic solution and a special paracervical block needle. There are several paracervical block needles including the Kobak needle, the Freeman needle, the Brittain needle and the Iowa trumpet. All have an outer guard or sheath which prevents the insertion of the inner needle for more than a few millimetres into the paracervical tissues. A paracervical block needle and the Iowa trumpet are illustrated in Figure 6.

With the patient in the dorsal position and after the usual antiseptic and aseptic preliminaries, the needle guard is pressed into the lateral fornix and the needle point is pushed into the paracervical tissues near the base of the broad ligament. The uterine artery lies close by and so only after careful aspiration for blood are 5 ml to 10 ml of local anaesthetic solution injected. The injection is repeated on the other side.

If 1 per cent lignocaine is used then analgesia lasts from 60 to 90 minutes and so repeated blocks will often be necessary. The agent of choice is bupivacaine (Marcain) in a 0.25 per cent solution. Analgesia with bupivacaine last for three hours on average. Prilocaine (Citanest) is better avoided for repeated blocks because of the likelihood of the development of methaemoglobinaemia.

Complications. The following complications may occur: Fetal bradycardia, intravascular injection, toxic reactions to the local anaesthetic, infection, failure of analgesia or unilateral analgesia.

An important complication is the frequent occurrence of fetal bradycardia. This slowing of the fetal heart rate is usually transient and is most likely to be observed within 20 minutes after injection. The cause of the fetal bradycardia is disputed and may be either an impairment of placental circulation or a depressant effect of the local anaesthetic drug on the fetal myocardium. According to some careful observers fetal bradycardia is detectable in over 30 per cent of cases. This bradycardia has been shown to be associated with a mild acidosis of the fetal scalp blood and so must be regarded as indicating at least a degree of fetal hypoxia. Of course other causes of fetal bradycardia must be considered when the fetal heart rate slows during paracervical block. Nevertheless it is probable that fetal death has been caused by paracervical block.

Paracervical block is a simple technique which can often give good analgesia when other methods of pain relief have proved inadequate. The availablity of bupivacaine has solved the problem of repeated injections and it is unfortunate that the frequent development of fetal bradycardia mars the safety of this otherwise valuable technique. The potential danger for the fetus and the wider availability of epidural analgesia have led most obstetricians to abandon the use of paracervical block.

Epidural analgesia

The terms extradural, epidural and peridural analgesia mean the same. The two forms of epidural analgesia used in obstetrics are lumbar epidural analgesia and caudal analgesia. Either may be used as a single injection ('single shot') or as a continuous technique, when a catheter is left in the epidural space. Top-up injections are given through the catheter and analgesia can be maintained for many hours.

Many maternity hospitals in the United Kingdom now make

regular use of continuous epidural analgesia for the relief of pain in the first stage of labour and single injection techniques are used for forceps delivery. A major restriction on the wider use of epidural analgesia is the absence of a resident anaesthetist in many maternity hospitals.

If the effects of epidural analgesia are to be understood it is necessary first to consider the nerve supply of the birth canal.

Sensory nerve supply of the birth canal

The body of the uterus. Sensation from the body of the uterus is transmitted by the paracervical plexus (ganglion) and various sympathetic pathways, to enter the spinal cord with the eleventh and twelfth thoracic nerves (T. 11 and 12) and probably also the first lumbar nerves (L. 1).

The cervix. Sensation from the cervix follows the above pathways and may also travel along the pelvic parasympathetic nerves (*nervi erigentes*) to enter the spinal cord at the 2nd, 3rd and 4th sacral segments (S. 2, 3 and 4). The existence of this second pathway is denied by some authorities.

The vagina, perineum and pelvic floor muscles. Sensation is transmitted mainly by the pudendal nerves and these nerves are also the motor nerves to the pelvic floor muscles. The roots of the pudendal nerves are in the 2nd, 3rd and 4th sacral segments of the spinal cord (S. 2, 3 and 4) (Fig. 7).

The abdominal cramping pains in the first stage of labour rise in body of the uterus and can be relieved by blocking T. 11 and 12 and L. 1 nerves. The backache which is often the most distressing feature of certain labours can sometimes be relieved by also blocking S. 2, 3 and 4 nerves. A painless forceps delivery can be performed after blocking these sacral nerves because the area supplied by the pudendal nerve will be analgesic.

An injection of an appropriate dose of local anaesthetic into the epidural space will block all the sacral, lumbar and lower thoracic nerves and relieve the pain of labour and delivery. The epidural injection may be performed in the lumbar region or through the sacrococcygeal membrane (caudal analgesia). The effects are essentially the same but many anaesthetists prefer the lumbar approach because it is nearly always successful and because a smaller dose of local anaesthetic is required.

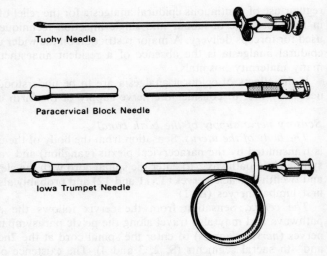

Fig. 6 Some needles used for regional analgesia.

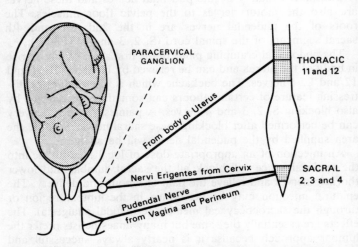

Fig. 7 Schematic representation of the sensory nerve supply of the birth canal.

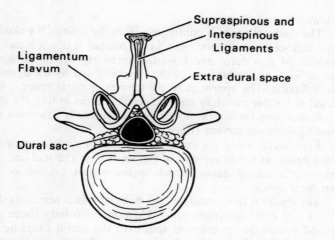

Fig. 8 Transverse section of a lumbar vertebra showing ligaments and epidural space.

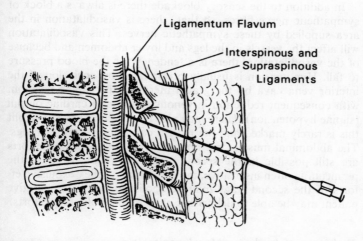

Fig. 9 Longitudinal section of lumbar spine showing ligaments and needle in the epidural space.

Anatomy and physiology

The epidural space is continuous from the base of the skull to the sacrococcygeal membrane. In the lumbar region it is narrow (about 4 mm deep) and bounded anteriorly by the dura and posteriorly by the laminae of the vertebrae and by the ligamentum flavum. The approach to the lumbar epidural space is that used in lumbar puncture and the needle pierces in turn the skin, subcutaneous fat, supraspinous and interspinous ligaments and the ligamentum flavum (Figs. 8 and 9).

For caudal analgesia the needle pierces the sacro-coccygeal membrane at the lower end of the sacrum in the mid-line and enters the sacral canal, which is the lowest portion of the epidural space.

The epidural space contains the pairs of spinal nerves as they leave and enter the spinal cord. There are also fatty tissue and blood vessels in the epidural space. In the sacral canal lie the nerves of the cauda equina. Local anaesthetics can spread freely in the epidural space and so can block the various spinal nerves. The extent of the spread depends on the dose of local anaesthetic injected.

In addition to the sensory blockade there is always a block of sympathetic nerve fibres, so that there is vasodilatation in the area supplied by these sympathetic nerves. This vasodilatation will affect the vessels in the legs and lower abdomen and because of the vasodilatation, there is a tendency for the blood pressure to fall. Hypotension is usually precipitated by occlusion of the inferior vena cava by the gravid uterus in the supine position, with consequent reduction in venous return and cardiac output (supine hypotension). There may also be muscular weakness, but this is rarely marked and the patient can usually move her legs. The abdominal muscles are not paralysed and expulsive efforts are still possible in the second stage of labour. Because the perineum is often insensitive, the involuntary, reflex expulsive efforts of the second stage may be abolished but a co-operative patient may be able to deliver her child by her voluntary efforts.

Technique of lumbar epidural analgesia

The patient sits on the edge of a tilting obstetric bed and rests her arms on the shoulders of an assistant who stands face to face with the patient. Alternatively the lateral lumbar puncture position may be used.

After a scrupulous antiseptic and aseptic preparation a little local anaesthetic solution is infiltrated into the skin and subcutaneous tissues at the L. 3–4 or L. 2–3 interspace. A 16 or 17 S.W.G. Tuohy needle is inserted so that its tip lies in the interspinous ligament. This needle has its opening at the side so that the passage of a plastic catheter is facilitated. A syringe of local anaesthetic solution, saline or air is now attached to the needle. The needle is advanced through the ligaments while a steady pressure is maintained on the plunger of the syringe. As the needle enters the epidural space there is a sensation of a sudden give and the injection of liquid or air is now very easy. This is the loss of resistance test and is a means of detecting the low or even sub-atmospheric pressure which exists in the epidural space. Some anaesthetists use various devices to detect this low pressure but probably none of these is as certain as the educated hand. Among the devices available are the Macintosh needle, the Macintosh balloon, the Ilke syringe and the Odom's indicator.

After careful aspiration for blood and for cerebrospinal fluid, the dose of local anaesthetic is injected and if a continuous technique is to be used then a plastic catheter is threaded through the needle. If top-up injections are to be given by a midwife, the anaesthetist injects the initial dose of local anaesthetic through the catheter and ensures that the catheter is correctly placed. The needle is withdrawn over the catheter and the catheter is attached to a sterile system which permits the injection of topping-up doses.

Suitable local anaesthetics are a 1.5 per cent or a 2 per cent solution of lignocaine to which adrenaline 1:200 000 has usually been added. Bupivacaine (Marcain) in 0.5 per cent or 0.25 per cent solution is often preferred because analgesia lasts longer with this agent.

The simplest topping-up system is a sterile 50 ml plastic syringe filled with sterile local anaesthetic solution and enclosed within a sterile transparent plastic bag. Many anaesthetists rely entirely upon a bacterial filter for sterility. Others prefer to use a sterile drip set connected to a sterile container of local anaesthetic solution. Whichever system is employed the use of a Millex (Millipore) filter is recommended, not only as a bacterial filter but also as a filter for minute particulate matter which might act as an irritant within the epidural space. Spicules of glass from ampoules, glove powder and fragments of foam rubber into which needles have been inserted have all been suggested as potential irritants. Usually top-up injections are given when pain returns and are required at intervals of from one and a half to four hours. The topping-up of epidural analgesia by midwives is discussed on page 92.

Technique of caudal analgesia

The injection may be made with the patient in the lateral, prone or knee-chest position. With the usual sterile technique a straight caudal needle some 8 to 10 cm long is inserted through the sacrococcygeal membrane and then advanced for 2 to 3 cm up the sacral canal. The site of injection is identified by feeling the sacral cornua, bony prominences on each side of the sacro-coccygeal membrane. Correct placement of the needle is confirmed by the ease with which local anaesthetic solution or air can be injected into the epidural space. Careful aspiration for blood and cerebrospinal fluid is carried out.

A dose of 20 to 30 ml of local anaesthetic solution is injected. Commonly used solutions are 1 per cent or 1.5 per cent lignocaine with 1:200 000 adrenaline and 0.25 per cent bupivacaine (Marcain).

A plastic catheter may be threaded through the needle for continuous caudal analgesia.

Puncture of the dura can occur with the lumbar and caudal approaches. The dural sac reaches down to the level of the second sacral foramen and so if the caudal needle or catheter is advanced too far up the sacral canal this complication may occur.

There is a failure rate of at least 10 per cent with caudal analgesia and the dose of local anaesthetic used is significantly greater than that required for lumbar analgesia. Some failures are unavoidable owing to the high incidence of abnormalities of the lower end of the sacrum.

The relaxation of the pelvic floor muscles which invariably accompanies caudal analgesia (but not lumbar epidural analgesia) may result in failure of rotation of the fetal head from its occipito-posterior position.

Complications of epidural analgesia. The incidence of complications varies with the experience of the anaesthetist and Table 4 indicates the approximate incidences of the various complications which may be expected in skilled hands. Lack of technical expertise by the anaesthetist and failure to provide close supervision in labour will increase the incidence of complications.

Table 4 Complications of Epidural Analgesia with Probable Incidence

	LUMBAR	CAUDAL
Hypotension (90 mm Hg (12 kPa systolic)	3 to 5%	2 to 5%
Toxic reactions	Almost none	1 to 4%
Total spinal anaesthesia	0.1%	0.1%
Dural tap (no injection)	1% to 2%	1%
Infection	None	None
Broken needle or catheter	Almost none	Almost none
Injection of fetus and fetal death	None	4 cases reported
Failure	2%	10% to 20%

Hypotension. The prevention and the initial treatment of hypotension are a legitimate concern of the midwife and hypotension is the commonest complication of epidural analgesia. There are two main causes of hypotension during epidural analgesia in labour and often both causes co-exist. Firstly the vasodilatation in the lower part of the body may cause pooling of the blood in the legs and lower abdomen and secondly the gravid uterus may compress the inferior vena cava when the patient lies on her back. Both of these factors predispose to pooling of blood in the veins of the legs and pelvis with a resulting reduction in the venous return to the heart, a lowered cardiac output and hypotension. It is important to realise that vena caval compression and the supine hypotensive syndrome which it may cause are often the precipitating cause of a fall in blood pressure during epidural analgesia. Hypovolaemia predisposes to serious hypotension during epidural analgesia.

The initial treatment of hypotension is to have the patient assume the left lateral position in order to relieve any obstruction of the inferior vena cava. It is also advisable, as far as possible, to encourage the patient to lie on her side during labour in order to prevent supine hypotension. In most cases the blood pressure will be restored to normal with this simple procedure, which should be carried out without sending for medical assistance. Should the use of the lateral position prove inadequate treatment, then the head of the bed should be lowered and oxygen administered. Treatment should be carried out if the blood pressure falls below 100 mmHg (13.3 kPa). Rarely an intravenous injection of a vasopressor drug such as ephedrine 10 mg will be required. The rapid intravenous infusion of 500 ml to 1000 ml of a crystoloid solution is often valuable. The use of the lateral position as advocated during labour may occasionally result in unilateral analgesia. This can be prevented by assuming alternately left and right lateral positions from time to time.

If the dorsal or lithotomy position is used for delivery, vaginal examination, catheterisation or fetal blood sampling then it is strongly recommended that the right buttock be elevated in order to rotate the uterus to the left. The Crawford wedge is available for this purpose. The progressive fetal acidosis which regularly occurs during the second stage of labour can be prevented by this simple procedure.

Total spinal anaesthesia. Total spinal anaesthesia occurs when a dose of local anaesthetic intended for the epidural space is accidentally injected into the subarachnoid space after undetected dural puncture. Because the dose of local anaesthetic drug is many times larger than that used for intentional spinal analgesia, a block of all the spinal nerves results. Within perhaps two minutes, spontaneous ventilation ceases and the blood pressure falls to very low levels. Treatment, which is the concern of the anaesthetist, consists essentially of immediate artificial ventilation, the injection of vasopressor drugs and the rapid infusion of fluids. The complication is rare but potentially fatal. With proper and rapid treatment, no harm should result.

Unblocked segment. With currently available local anaesthetic drugs one or more spinal nerves will be unaffected in from 4 per cent to 7 per cent of patients. Most often there is persistent pain in one groin during an otherwise successful block. Sometimes a further injection of 3 ml or 4 ml of solution will be effective if given while the patient lies on the painful side. Carbonated local anaesthetics were said to avoid this complication but in a controlled trial were found to be ineffective.

Unilateral block. In this situation analgesia is entirely absent on one side. Pain is usually felt on the uppermost side when the patient has been in the lateral position and is relieved by giving a top-up injection while the mother lies on the painful side. A contributory cause may be the insertion of more than 2–3 cm of catheter into the epidural space.

Headache and backache. An uncomplicated epidural block does not cause headache. A 'spinal' headache is likely to develop about 24 hours after a dural puncture and may be effectively treated by epidural saline injection, or by the injection of 10 ml to 20 ml of the patient's own blood into the epidural space to form a 'blood patch'. A spinal headache is due to the leakage of cerebro-spinal fluid through the dural puncture and both the foregoing treatments arrest this leakage. When the dura has been punctured the patient should remain in bed for at least 24 hours and she should lie in the prone (face-down) position as much as possible. The incidence of headache and backache was no different in a series of forceps deliveries performed under epidural and pudendal nerve block.

The other complications listed in Table 4 need not be discussed here. Although they make an impressive list, many are rare and not all present a risk to life. In practice, epidural analgesia has been shown to be safer than general anaesthesia in several series of many thousands of cases but it is not a technique for the inexperienced doctor or the inadequately staffed hospital.

The management of labour during epidural analgesia

It is assumed that the normal routine care of a patient in labour will be carried out. The following points are directly related to the use of epidural analgesia.

Blood pressure recording. Hypotension is more likely to occur shortly after an injection but may occur at any time. It is recommended that the blood pressure be recorded every 5 minutes for 20 minutes after each injection and thereafter every 15 minutes.

Should the systolic pressure fall below 100 mm Hg (13.3 kPa) the patient should immediately be turned on to her left side. This will usually be effective but if the blood pressure is not restored to at least 100 mm Hg (13.3kPa) then the head of the bed should be lowered and oxygen administered. It is of course, preferrable to prevent caval occlusion by nursing all patients in the lateral or tilted position. On the rare occasion when these simple measures are ineffective then medical aid should be summoned. If an intravenous infusion is running then the rapid administration of 500 ml of fluid may raise the blood pressure. The anaesthetist may administer an intravenous injection of ephedrine 5 mg to 15 mg and this drug should always be readily available.

As far as possible the patient should lie on her side during labour and she should not get out of bed because disastrous hypotension may develop in the erect position. Nausea, retching, palor, dizziness or sweating may be indications of hypotension. Hypotension is dangerous for the mother and the fetus. If the maternal blood pressure falls below 80 mm Hg then the placental circulation may be inadequate for fetal oxygenation.

Top-up injections. The Central Midwives Board for England and Wales has recently approved the administration of top-up injections by experienced midwives and has issued the following statement of policy. 'The Board would raise no objection to an experienced midwife undertaking the topping-up procedure (not the primary dose through the catheter) in the maintenance of an epidural block provided the following safeguards are observed:

a. that the ultimate responsibility for such a technique should be clearly stated to rest with the doctor;

b. that written instructions as to the dose should be given by the doctor concerned;

c. that in all cases the dose given by the midwife should be checked by one other person;

d. that instructions should be given by the doctor as to the posture of the patient at the time of injection, observation of blood pressure etc., and measures to be taken in the event of any side effect;

e. that the midwife should have been thoroughly instructed in the technique so that the doctor concerned is satisfied as to her ability'.

These recommendations should help to make epidural analgesia more widely available, especially in hospitals with a numerically small medical staff. Active involvement in epidural analgesia is usually welcomed by midwives whose role is thereby extended. The C.M.B. for Scotland has not yet sanctioned the giving of top-up injections by midwives, but is actively considering this measure.

The technique used will vary at the discretion of the anaesthetist and it is not possible to describe all the methods used. Probably the two most popular methods are the use of a sterile 50 ml syringe within a sterile plastic bag and injection through a Millipore (Millex) filter on the proximal end of the catheter.

The bladder. Because the bladder may be insensitive during epidural analgesia, retention of urine may cause no discomfort. It is important to watch for the signs of retention of urine and if necessary to empty the bladder by passing a catheter. Retention of urine (sometimes painless) and difficulty in initiating the flow of urine are common in the early puerperium, but these difficulties are also seen where epidural analgesia has not been used and are more likely to be due to instrumental delivery or prolonged labour, than to epidural block.

Uterine contractions. Epidural analgesia has no significant effect on the uterine contractions of established normal labour and may be followed by a more normal type of uterine activity if inco-ordinate uterine action exists. It is important to rely on abdominal palpation or a recorder to assess the strength of the contractions and to beware of thinking that the intensity of the contractions has been reduced because the patient's response to the now painless contractions has been abolished by epidural analgesia.

Continuous monitoring of the fetal heart rate and uterine contractions is of great value and an automatic blood pressure recorder such as the Arteriosonde has been helpful. It may be advisable to perform vaginal examinations according to a schedule because it is sometimes difficult to estimate progress by other means.

Four hourly intervals between examinations are sometimes advocated and if labour is being accelerated then two hourly intervals may be appropriate. Descent of the fetal head into the pelvis may indicate the onset of the second stage. It is important that full dilatation of the cervix should not go undetected in the patient in whom anaesthesia has abolished involuntary expulsive efforts.

Severe hypotension may temporarily abolish uterine contractions because of the reduction in myometrial blood flow. Uterine action should be restored when hypotension has been corrected. The active management of labour with controlled and escalating dosage of Syntocinon and intensive monitoring of uterine action and the fetal heart rate lends itself admirably to the use of epidural analgesia. Accelerated and painless labour has revolutionised labour room practice in a growing number of hospitals. Although accelerated labours may diminish mental distress and the physical side-effects of, prolonged labour (tachycardia, pyrexia, ketosis and dehydration) are now rare, accelerated labours may be acutely painful and effective analgesia is required. In some hospitals epidural analgesia is initiated at the time of amniotomy.

Intravenous fluids. Most patients receiving epidural analgesia are likely to benefit from an intravenous infusion. Hypotension is less likely to develop if an adequate circulating blood volume is maintained. It is good practice to have an intravenous infusion running during every epidural block and most certainly an intravenous needle or cannula should be in place.

Oxytocic drug at delivery. About 40 per cent of the patients who receive an intravenous injection of ergometrine at delivery under epidural analgesia experience retching or vomiting. Hypertension and a rise in central venous pressure are also common. It is the writer's opinion that an intravenous injection of 5 or 10 units of oxytocin (Syntocinon) should be substituted for ergometrine.

Top-up injections. These are given when pain returns. Unilateral analgesia sometimes develops during labour. This can usually be rectified by injecting a further 3 ml or 4 ml of solution while the patient lies on the unaffected side. Unilateral analgesia may be prevented by injecting half of the dose while the patient lies on her side and injecting the remainder of the dose 10 minutes later while the patient lies on her other side. Unilateral analgesia also results from the insertion of an excessive length of catheter. If perineal analgesia is required then the injection may be made while the patient sits up.

Indications for epidural analgesia

Continuous epidural analgesia is the most effective method of pain relief available for use in labour and so may be used for any patient who is not receiving adequate analgesia from more conventional methods. There are also certain abnormal situations in which epidural analgesia may be of value, not only for the pain relief obtained but also for its effects on uterine action or for its hypotensive effect. In any situation where respiratory depressant drugs are particularly dangerous, then epidural analgesia may be used.

In prolonged labour associated with inco-ordinate uterine action, it has been found that in over 70 per cent of patients there was a substantial increase in the rate of cervical dilatation after instituting epidural analgesia. It is likely that Caesarean section can sometimes be avoided in patients with inco-ordinate uterine action and it is therefore especially valuable in the younger primigravida. The relief of pain and distress is dramatic and Caesarean section need not be performed primarily for the relief of intolerable distress. The perinatal mortality is not increased when epidural analgesia is used in inco-ordinate uterine action. Of course when cephalopelvic disproportion or fetal distress is associated with inco-ordinate uterine action, Caesarean section may still be necessary. The combination of epidural analgesia and intravenous Syntocinon is particularly effective in managing inco-ordinate labour.

When severe hypertension is present during labour, a useful reduction in blood pressure can usually be obtained with epidural block and the administration of large doses of depressant drugs is unnecessary. The further rises in blood pressure which usually accompany painful uterine contractions are abolished.

A single injection into the epidural space provides excellent conditions for forceps delivery and avoids the risks of general anaesthesia for mother and fetus. Epidural analgesia can be used for Caesarean section. Although the idea of undergoing abdominal surgery while conscious is alarming to many women, the reward of being awake at the birth of the child can make it a worthwhile experience. Here again the very real risks of general asaesthesia can be avoided. Epidural analgesia far from being contraindicated for breech delivery is now regarded as the method of choice if vaginal delivery is to be permitted. Although the second stage is slightly prolonged the controlled and painless delivery is associated with demonstrable improvement in the condition of the infant.

The indications for epidural analgesia are listed in Table 5.

Table 5 Indications for Epidural Analgesia in Obsterics

Severe pain in labour.
Inco-ordinate uterine action.
Hypertension in labour.
Patients with cardiac and respiratory
    disease in labour.
Forceps delivery
Caesarean section
Breech delivery.

These are the now quite widely accepted indications for epidural analgesia, and in hospitals where they are observed an epidural analgesia rate of about 25 per cent is likely. In a few hospitals epidural analgesia is offered to all primigravidae and then some 60 to 70 per cent of patients may receive an epidural block. The condition of newborn infants in comparable series is consistently better when delivery takes place under epidural analgesia in contrast with pethidine analgesia or general anaesthesia. This statement can be confirmed by Apgar scores, measurement of acid-base status and by the sensitive techniques of neuro-behavioural assessment.

Spinal (subarachnoid) analgesia

This technique is seldom used today in the United Kingdom, although it is extensively used in many other countries.

A single injection of local anaesthetic solution into the subarachnoid space can provide excellent analgesia for forceps delivery. Hyperbaric solutions are usually preferred. These are solutions of local anaesthetic drug dissolved in 6 per cent glucose so that their specific gravity is greater than that of the cerebrospinal fluid. The local anaesthetic solution tracks downwards under the influence of gravity when the patient is appropriately positioned. A small dose of local anaesthetic injected in the lumbar region while the patient sits upright will give analgesia of the sacral nerve roots only and hypotension is unlikely. This technique is sometimes called saddleblock analgesia and is suitable for forceps delivery. Spinal analgesia may be used for Caesarean section but then the analgesia must extend up to the lower thoracic nerve roots and the risk of sudden profound hypotension is considerable and maternal deaths have occurred from this cause. Continuous spinal analgesia is no longer used.

The complications of spinal analgesia are similar to those of epidural analgesia but hypotension may develop more rapidly. An important complication of subarachnoid analgesia is post-lumbar puncture headache. This may be very distressing and may last for several days. The incidence of headache may be as high as 40 per cent if large needles are used and can be reduced to about 5 per cent by using fine needles (22 or 24 S.W.G.) and to one per cent with 25 S.W.G. needles. Very rarely damage to the central nervous system has followed spinal analgesia and has caused permanent paraplegia. This dreadful complication was probably due to chemical contamination of the local anaesthetic solution from the now utterly condemned practice of storing the ampoules in solutions of phenol.

It is the incidence of hypotension and headache and the probably exaggerated fear of neurological complications which have led to the near abandonment of spinal analgesia in the United Kingdom. Although spinal analgesia is a potentially dangerous anaesthetic for Caesarean section, it is perhaps unfortunate that it has been almost abandoned for forceps delivery. Hopefully a modest revival is taking place in a few centres.

Preparation of equipment for regional analgesia

Because each obstetrician and anaesthetist will have his own preferences for needles, syringes and local anaesthetic drugs and each hospital will have its own procedures for sterilisation, it is only possible to offer some guidance on the preparation of equipment.

It is of course mandatory that every piece of equipment be sterile. The basic tray of syringes, gallipots and drapes must be autoclaved.

For epidural and subarachnoid analgesia the local anaesthetic solutions must be autoclaved. The local anaesthetics are for practical purposes unaffected even by repeated autoclaving. Occasionally, inactivation of adrenaline has been observed after exposure to the high temperatures reached in modern autoclaves and then a brown or pink colour may develop. This alteration is in itself harmless but of course the adrenaline will no longer be effective. A sterile file may be needed for opening ampoules of local anaesthetic. It is quite wrong to draw up local anaesthetic solution from an ampoule whose contents may be sterile but whose exterior is unsterile. After autoclaving, local anaesthetic solutions containing dextrose may turn brown. This is due to caramelisation of the sugar and is harmless.

Needles should be sterilised in a hot air oven although autoclaving is accepted as adequate by many. Disposable needles are generally preferred.

For epidural and subarachnoid blocks glass syringes are preferred by many anaesthetists. Before autoclaving, these syringes should be washed out with water. A detergent should not be used for this purpose. Damage to nerve tissues has been attributed to the contamination of syringes or needles with traces of detergent.

Ampoules of local anaesthetic must never be stored in antiseptic solutions. The antiseptic solution has been shown to be able to penetrate microscopic cracks in the ampoules and strong antiseptics such as phenol can destroy nerve tissue.

Plastic catheters for continuous epidural analgesia are usually obtained presterilised by the manufacturers. Where the syringe-in-bag method is used for continuous epidural analgesia plastic bags may be made from suitable lengths of transparent plastic sleeving which have been heat-sealed at one end. These bags are then autoclaved.

Presterilised disposable needles for spinal, and caudal analgesia are now available in the United Kingdom. Several disposable sets for epidural analgesia are now marketed. Although their contents are not always entirely to the liking of the individual anaesthetist their introduction is, on balance to be welcomed.

7. General Anaesthesia, Resuscitation and the Unconscious Patient

General anaesthesia

In Great Britain general anaesthesia is now administered almost exclusively by specialist anaesthetists. Even so, every member of the obstetric team is involved to some extent in the preparation for anaesthesia and in post-operative care and should have some knowledge of the special problems and risks of general anaesthesia in obstetrics.

There has recently been a most disturbing increase in the percentage of British mothers whose deaths have been caused by the complications of general anaesthesia. For many years some 4 per cent of maternal deaths had been caused by anaesthesia. The percentage has now recently more than doubled and this has occurred at a time when maternal deaths from almost every other cause have decreased in number. In 1970–1972 in England and Wales, 10.4 per cent of all maternal deaths were associated with complications of anaesthesia. The increased anaesthetic mortality is due to a sharp rise in the number of deaths from Mendelson's syndrome and to hypoxia which is often the result of difficult or failed intubation of the trachea.

Mendelson's syndrome

Mendelson's syndrome, also known as the acid-aspiration syndrome, is caused by the entry of highly acid gastric juice into the lungs during general anaesthesia. The chemical irritation set up by the hydrochloric acid causes a tremendous outpouring of fluid into the alveoli. Cyanosis, tachycardia, bronchospasm, hypotension and cardiac failure may all occur. Death, if it occurs, may be delayed for some hours or days. This dreadful condition does not occur in a severe form unless the gastric juice which is aspirated into the lungs is very acid (pH under 2.5). Consequently Mendelson's syndrome can be prevented by rendering the stomach contents less acid by the administration of oral antacids before general anaesthesia. There is good reason to believe that if an appropriate dietary regime is combined with the administration of alkalis to women in labour then deaths from Mendelson's syndrome would not occur.

Diet in labour

A dietary regime for patients in labour should be designed to prevent acute asphyxial deaths from the aspiration of solid food into the lungs and deaths from Mendelson's syndrome caused by the aspiration of highly acid gastric juice.

The practice in the Queen Mother's Hospital, Glasgow, is to give no solid food to patients in labour. Intravenous fluids are almost always administered and the deprivation of oral sustenance causes little hardship during the short labours which are usually achieved with the help of intravenous Syntocinon. The measures taken to prevent Mendelson's syndrome are the two hourly administration of 15 ml of magnesium trisilicate to every patient in active labour. An additional 30 ml dose of this antacid is given immediately before the administration of a general anaesthetic. 0.3 molar sodium citrate has been used as an antacid prior to anaesthesia for patients who had not received magnesium trisilicate in labour, but evaluation on a large scale is awaited.

It should be appreciated that dietary restriction and antacid therapy are both essential. If a patient is starved, but does not receive an alkali then she is quite likely to have a small quantity of very acid juice in her stomach and the stage is set for the development of Mendelson's syndrome.

Emptying the stomach

In order to empty the stomach before general anaesthesia the anaesthetist may order a stomach tube to be passed. An oesophageal tube should be used. A Ryle's tube is too small to be useful. Gastric intubation is perhaps less frequently used now because a stomach tube does not always empty the stomach, although it will usually remove some liquid and gas and by reducing the intragastric pressure may lessen the risk of regurgitation of stomach contents. A few anaesthetists administer apomorphine intravenously in order to induce vomiting before anaesthesia. Although this procedure is claimed to be slightly less unpleasant than gastric intubation, neither of these techniques can ensure an empty stomach. Nevertheless the reduction of intra-gastric pressure may be valuable.

The gastric emptying time is prolonged in many patients in labour. Sedative and analgesic drugs contribute to the tendency to retain food in the stomach for many hours. Although metoclopramide (Maxolon) can sometimes accelerate gastric emptying it is probably ineffective when delay is due to narcotic analgesics.

The use of regional analgesia in preference to general anaesthesia, especially for forceps deliveries, is an obvious way to avoid the greatest hazard of general anaesthesia in obstetrics, death of the mother from the aspiration of stomach contents into the lungs. Hiatus hernia is relatively common in pregnancy, as is heartburn. Patients with these conditions are especially liable to regurgitate stomach contents under anaesthesia, with consequent risk of aspiration of these stomach contents into the lungs.

A policy of food and fluid restriction must entail the more liberal use of intravenous fluids if the patient is not to be deprived of water, electrolytes and calories during labour lasting for more than a few hours.

Intravenous fluid therapy

The normal adult requires an intake of about 3 litres of fluid in 24 hours. A woman in labour requires substantially more than this if she is to make up for extra loss by vomiting and in the expired air if she is hyperventilating. Calorie requirements must also be met and ketonuria (acetonuria) in labour is common and is an indication for intravenous sugar solutions.

For maintenance therapy, electrolytes and water can be supplied by normal saline solution, or better by a balanced salt solution such as Ringer's or Hartman's solutions. These last solutions contain sodium, potassium and chloride in approximately the concentrations present in normal plasma. This is not the case with normal saline which contains an excess of chloride ions. Calories are supplied by 5 per cent or 10 per cent dextrose (glucose) solutions. A 20 per cent solution of laevulose (fructose) provides more calories than dextrose solutions and is useful for the rapid correction of ketonuria. Dextrose causes venous thrombosis when administered in concentrations greater than 10 per cent. A commercial preparation known as Plasmalyte supplies water, electrolytes and calories in a single bottle and is convenient for maintenance therapy. Ketonuria and dehydration are now more rare thanks to shorter labours and routine intravenous fluid therapy.

Premedication

Premedication may be given in order (1) to relieve anxiety, (2) to relieve pain if it is present, (3) to prevent excessive salivation and the formation of tracheo-bronchial secretions and (4) to prevent dangerous cardiac arrythmias, including excessive slowing of the heart rate and cardiac arrest.

Unfortunately the drugs used in premedication cross the placental barrier freely and so many anaesthetists do not prescribe sedative or analgesic drugs before elective Caesarean section. Others prescribe small doses of tranquillising drugs. Analgesics are, of course, not required before an elective Caesarean section. Patients in labour will often have received sedatives and analgesics earlier in the course of labour.

Atropine 0.6 mg is often given by intramuscular injection to prevent salivation and to dry up secretions in the respiratory tract. Atropine may be given intravenously to prevent undue slowing of the heart rate during anaesthesia. Scopolamine (hyoscine) 0.4 mg is a better drying agent than atropine and also has a sedative action. Scopolamine is sometimes given intravenously by the anaesthetist to reduce the incidence of awareness during anaesthesia.

Patients often welcome anaesthesia at the end of a long labour and their attitude is rather different from that of a patient who is about to undergo elective surgery for a serious illness. There is also much truth in the statement that a sympathetic nurse is worth more than any premedication.

Other preparations for anaesthesia

The patient's identity should be checked verbally and from her name band. Dentures and dental plates, watches and jewellery should be removed. The wedding ring, if retained, should be covered with adhesive tape. The bowel and bladder should be empty if possible, but an enema is not usually indicated. The obstetrician may wish to catheterise the bladder himself. Cross-matched blood should be available, preferably in the operating theatre, for Caesarean sections and the identity of the bottle or bag should be carefully checked. A blood warmer should be available.

The patient should be on a tilting bed or operating table. The Steel and the Oxford obstetric beds are very suitable and can with benefit be used for all patients in labour, thus avoiding the need to transfer the patient to another bed for delivery under anaesthesia. It is recommended that patients should assume the left lateral position for some 15 minutes before anaesthesia. This should prevent occlusion of the inferior vena cava by the gravid uterus with the attendant risks of reducing utero-placental blood flow for the fetus. It is believed that placental blood flow may be impaired even in the absence of overt supine hypotension. Many anaesthetists now induce anaesthesia with the patient tilted slightly towards the left. In the absence of a laterally tilting table a rubber wedge may be placed under the right buttock and thorax. A wedge should also be used whenever a patient is in the lithotomy position.

Special categories of patient will require special preparations. The diabetic patient should receive her insulin in the form of soluble insulin and her calorie requirements should be supplied by an intravenous dextrose (glucose) infusion. Oral glucose solutions should never be given before general anaesthesia. Patients who have received a course of steroid hormone therapy within recent months may be given intramuscular injections of hydrocortisone before and after operation to prevent collapse during anaesthesia. Hydrocortisone hemisuccinate may be given intravenously during anaesthesia if collapse occurs.

The anaesthetist should be informed if the patient has used a Trilene inhaler during labour so that he may avoid the use of soda lime.

The anaesthetic

The special problems of obstetric anaesthesia are:

1. The high risk of the aspiration of stomach contents into the lungs causing death of the mother.

2. The free placental transfer of all anaesthetic drugs (except the muscle relaxants) which may affect the newborn.

3. The depressant effect of anaesthetics on uterine tone which may cause haemorrhage in the third stage.

4. The liability to hypotension caused by the anaesthetic, compression of the inferior vena cava or haemorrhage.

5. The need for relaxation of the abdominal or pelvic floor muscles.

6. The necessity for the anaesthetist to resuscitate the baby and maintain anaesthesia simultaneously in many hospitals.

7. The need to ensure unconsciousness and yet to administer the lightest possible anaesthetic.

8. The harmful effect of any mishap is often more serious for the fetus than the mother.

The technique of general anaesthesia used by most British anaesthetists is fairly standardised and is designed, as far as possible, to take account of the various special problems of the obstetric patient. Compromises are necessary. For example, the anaesthetic should be kept very light for the sake of the baby and to minimise bleeding. Because of this the patient may sometimes be too lightly anaesthetised and may be aware of her surroundings at least during some part of the anaesthetic. Using unsupplemented nitrous oxide and oxygen anaesthesia, up to 8 per cent of patients have been found to have some definite memory of events which occurred during Caesarean section. Analgesic levels of nitrous oxide may prevent appreciation of pain, but the experience is distressing.

A widely used technique of anaesthesia is as follows:

30 ml of magnesium trisilicate are given by mouth and atropine 0.6 mg is given by intramuscular or intravenous injection.

A needle is inserted into a vein or an intravenous infusion is set up. The patient breathes oxygen for three minutes (preoxygenation). The midwife may be asked to administer the oxygen.

Anaesthesia is rapidly induced with thiopentone (Pentothal), methohexitone (Brietal) or propanidid (Epontol) followed by suxamenthonium (Scoline). The new steriod anaesthetic Althesin has been successfully used to induce anaesthesia for obstetric operations.

Many anaesthetists use cricoid pressure (Sellick's manoeuvre) during intubation and the midwife may be asked to carry out this procedure. The tip of the thumb and the index finger are placed over the cricoid cartilage, which can be felt as a hard knob immediately below the thyroid cartilage (Adam's apple). The cricoid cartilage is pressed backwards so that the oesophagus is compressed between the cartilage and the vertebral column, thus preventing stomach contents from emerging from the oesophagus.

When a cuffed endotracheal tube has been inserted, anaesthesia is maintained with nitrous oxide and oxygen which may be supplemented with minimal concentrations of halothane (Fluothane), trichloroethylene (Trilene), or methoxyflurance (Penthrane) to ensure unconsciousness. Muscular relaxation is maintained with further doses of a muscle relaxant and intermittent positive pressure ventilation is performed by hand or with a ventilator.

The midwife can help the anaesthetist by understanding his needs and ensuring that equipment is in working order. In particular the anaesthetist will require an efficient suction apparatus, a laryngoscope and cuffed endotracheal tubes. The midwife who is assisting the anaesthetist should not leave his side without permission. The induction of anaesthesia is the most dangerous part of most obstetric operations and the anaesthetist may require immediate assistance. Maternal hypoxia or hypotension may kill the fetus while leaving the mother unharmed. The hypoxia which may result from failure to intubate the trachea has caused several maternal deaths in recent years.

Ketamine (Ketalar). This relatively new anaesthetic agent is given by intravenous or intramuscular injection. Ketamine produces unconsciousness associated with profound analgesia. Hypertension may occur and ketamine is usually avoided in pre-eclampsia. Ketamine has been used in conjunction with a muscle relaxant for Caesarean sections and it is possible to perform forceps delivery under ketamine alone. The technique is simple but not entirely free of risk. Most British anaesthetists prefer more sophisticated techniques. Ketamine has proved useful when tracheal intubation has been impossible or when the anaesthetist is unskilled in intubation.

The unconscious patient

The most important single aspect of the nursing care of the unconscious patient is the maintenance of a clear airway.

Care of the airway. The common causes of obstruction of the upper air passages in the unconscious patient are: (1) The tongue falling back on to the posterior wall of the pharynx.

2. The presence of vomitus, blood or mucus in the throat.

3. Laryngeal spasm.

Respiratory obstruction kills many unconscious patients and contributes to the deaths of others. The signs of upper airway obstruction are cyanosis, forcible movements of the chest wall which fail to move air in and out of the lungs and noisy breathing if the obstruction is incomplete. A stertorous, snoring noise suggests that the tongue has fallen back and a high-pitched crowing noise suggests laryngeal spasm. If respiratory obstruction is complete, there will be no noise. 'Noisy breathing is obstructed breathing but not all obstructed breathing is noisy.'

Treatment of airway obstruction. The treatment is essentially the same whatever the cause of the obstruction.

1. Lift the tongue forwards by pulling on the point of the chin, or by inserting a finger behind the angle of each jaw, just below the ear lobes and lifting the jaw forwards.

2. Suck out any foreign material from the throat and nose.

3. Administer oxygen.

4. If these measures are not quickly successful send for help.

The safest position for the unconscious patient is the lateral position. If unconsciousness is prolonged then the patient should be turned on the to the opposite side at two hourly intervals to reduce the risk of developing pneumonia.

The midwife may have to care for patients who are unconscious after general anaesthesia, eclampsia or the drugs given for the prevention and treatment of eclampsia and miscellaneous non-obstetric conditions.

Other aspects: The unconscious or anaesthetised patient may suffer injuries because she is deprived of the protective mechanism of pain. Great care must be observed when turning unconscious patients. Fractures may occur. An unnatural position of the limb is likely to be a dangerous position.

In the operating theatre prolonged pressure may damage nerves. Commoner causes of this type of paralysis are pressure against lithotomy poles which should be padded or kept away from the legs, pressure of shoulder rests against the brachial plexus in the neck (a non-slip mattress is preferable to shoulder rests), pressure on the radial nerve in the upper arm and the ulnar nerve at the point of the elbow. The brachial plexus may be injured by incorrect positioning of the arm on an arm board. The arm should not be abducted through more than 90 degrees and should not be forced downwards below the mid-axillary line.

The hands of the unconscious patient should not be placed under her buttocks.

Aspects of resuscitation

Only a few particular aspects of the resuscitation of the obstetric patient can be considered in a book such as this. The topics chosen are all fundamental and some of them involve the consideration of relatively new and difficult fields of knowledge. Some of the subects are outwith the province of treatment which a midwife might undertake, but they are included in order to try to offer a simplified explanation of complex and important subjects.

Cardiac and respiratory arrest

Cardiac arrest is usually swiftly followed by respiratory arrest and so treatment usually involves the maintenance of circulation and respiration by artificial means.

Cardiac arrest is uncommon in obstetric patients but treatment is more likely to be successful in a fundamentally healthy young mother than in an ill and elderly patient. The treatment of cardiac arrest must be undertaken without hesitation by whoever is present at the time. If an adequate circulation is not restored within three minutes then irreversible brain damage is likely to occur. If, as is often the case, the patient has suffered from hypoxia and a failing circulation before the cardiac arrest then the brain may not survive undamanged for as long as three minutes.

Every midwife should be familiar with the treatment of cardiac arrest and must be prepared to act immediately.

The diagnosis of cardiac arrest. If the pulses cannot be felt and if respirations have ceased the diagnosis must be presumed to be that of cardiac arrest and treatment must be instituted without delay. Absence of the carotid artery pulse in the neck is particularly significant because the radial pulses may be impalpable in the shocked patient who has not had a cardiac arrest. The patient may be pale and cyanosed. The pupils are commonly widely dilated. Consciousness is lost.

The treatment of cardio-respiratory arrest. The two essentials are external cardiac massage and artificial ventilation of the lungs.

External cardiac massage: If circumstances permit then place the patient on a hard surface such as the floor or insert a board under the mattress. Cardiac massage is more effective on a hard surface. Place the palm of one hand over the lower part of the sternum. Place the other hand on top of the first hand and press the 'heel' of the upper hand sharply downwards on to the lower hand. Repeat this motion about 60 times per minute. The heart will be intermittently compressed between the sternum and the vertebral column, achieving an artificial pumping action. Allow time for the heart to fill with blood between compressions and resist the temptation to massage very rapidly. Successful massage will produce palpable carotid pulses, the skin colour will improve and the pupils will become smaller.

There is no place for opening the chest and performing internal cardiac massage in the first aid treatment of cardiac arrest. This statement contradicts older teachings which encouraged this dramatic action.

Artificial respiration: The only worthwhile forms of artificial respiration are those which involve intermittent positive pressure ventilation (I.P.P.V.) The simplest of these methods and one which is always available is expired air resuscitation (mouth to mouth breathing, the kiss of life).

To perform expired air resuscitation, first ensure that the airway is clear. Hold the chin forward and remove any foreign material from the throat with a suction apparatus or with the finger. Unless the airway is patent artificial ventilation cannot succeed. Next, pinch the patient's nostrils with the other hand and place your lips over the patient's lips, making an airtight seal. Blow into the patient's mouth. The chest should expand. Now remove your lips from the patient and allow her to exhale passively. Repeat the manoeuvre 10 to 15 times per minute.

Expired-air resusciation can maintain life but there are improvements in this method which should be used if available. The Brook and Safar airways help to keep the tongue forwards and avoid the necessity for direct contact with the patient's lips which some find unaesthetic. The Ambu and similar bag and mask resuscitators are valuable. They consist of a face mask, a one-way valve and a self-expanding bag which fills with air. The mask must be fitted closely to the face, precisely in the manner used for administering inhalational analgesia and the bag is then squeezed intermittently. A flow of oxygen not exceeding 4 litres per minute may be run into the Ambu bag.

It will be apparent that one person cannot efficiently perform external cardiac massage and intermittent positive pressure ventilation at the same time. Where two persons undertake the resuscitation, one individual should perform 8 or 10 cardiac compressions and should then pause to allow the other person to inflate the lungs once or twice. This cycle is repeated until resuscitation is successful or is abandoned. If the midwife is alone she should summon assistance and meanwhile must do her best to perform cardiac massage and artificial ventilation alternately.

These techniques can be practised in the classroom on one of the model patients available for this purpose.

Other measures: The following resuscitative measures are the concern of the medical staff and are of secondary important to the performance of external cardiac massage and artificial ventilation of the lungs. Sodium bicarbonate solution may be given intravenously to counteract the metabolic acidosis which develops after circulatory arrest. An 8.4 per cent solution of sodium bicarbonate is commonly used and up to 200 ml may be injected. An endotracheal tube may be passed and intermittent positive pressure ventilation continued with oxygen. Other drugs which may be injected intravenously or into the heart include adrenaline 1:10 000, isoprenaline 0.01 mg/ml and calcium chloride (or gluconate) in 1 per cent solution.

An electro-cardiograph will be necessary to distinguish between cardiac arrest (asystole) and ventricular fibrillation. If ventricular fibrillation is present then an electric defibrillator will be required. Defibrillation will usually be attempted by the application of the electrodes to the chest wall and delivering one or more electric shocks. Should external defibrillation prove unsuccessful a thoracotomy may be performed to allow internal defibrillation by applying an electric shock directly to the heart. A direct current defibrillator is now preferred to the older alternating current apparatus.

Shock

The common feature in almost all shocked patients is a reduction in the circulating blood volume which usually results in a fall in blood pressure, a rise in pulse rate and a poor circulation. Shock in obstetric patients is usually due to blood loss but may also be caused by an excessive loss of body fluids through vomiting or diarrhoea. The presence of bacteria and their toxins in the blood stream can cause bacteraemic or endotoxic shock and may complicate abortion, surgery and even catheterisation of the bladder.

If the midwife is to offer the maximum of assistance in the treatment of shock she must have an understanding of the various diagnostic and resuscitative measures which may be used and for this reason the following outlines of some important concepts and recent developments in this field are offered.

The pulse rate and blood pressure. Although classically the pulse rate rises and the arterial blood pressure falls after the loss of blood or other body fluids, these changes are not completely reliable. A healthy young adult may lose more than a litre of blood and still maintain a normal pulse rate and blood pressure and this situation is common in obstetric patients. Such a patient may be on the brink of serious collapse. Quite moderate further bleeding may result in sudden severe hypotension and if general anaesthesia is induced, the associated vasodilatation may interfere with compensatory mechanisms and cause circulatory collapse. Consequently, whenever possible, patients who have experienced even moderately severe haemorrhage should be transfused with blood or other appropriate fluid before anaesthesia and surgery.

The skin in shock. The state of the peripheral circulation can be assessed by the condition of the skin. If the skin is cold and pale and the lips and nailbeds are cyanosed, then the peripheral circulation is inadequate. If the skin is warm and pink and the circulation returns rapidly following the temporary blanching produced by a brief pressure with the thumb, then the peripheral circulation is good, even if the blood pressure is low. This is sometimes the situation during epidural block and provides confirmation that the blood pressure is not by itself a sufficient guide to the adequacy or otherwise of the circulation. The gradient between the skin temperature (for example at the great toe) and the rectal or oesophageal temperature is a useful indicator of the peripheral circulation. The larger the gradient, the poorer is the peripheral circulation.

The central venous pressure. The central venous pressure is the pressure of the blood within the subclavian vein, the superior vena cava or the right atrium of the heart. The pressure is the same in all these situations because there are no intervening valves.

In clinical practice the central venous pressure (C. V. P.) is usually measured by inserting a long C. V. P. cannula from an elbow vein or the external jugular vein into the subclavian vein or the superior vena cava. The cannula is connected to an infusion set which has a simple liquid manometer incorporated to enable the C. V. P. to be recorded. When the cannula is correctly placed the liquid in the manometer pulsates with each heart beat and the level fluctuates with each breath. Before taking a C. V. P. reading the zero mark on the manometer scale must be level with either the manubrio-sternal junction or the mid-axillary line. The normal C. V. P. lies between zero and 3 cm water (0.5 kPa) measured from the manubrio-sternal junction and from 5–10 cm water (0.9 to 1.8 kPa) measured from the mid-axillary line).

Monitoring the C. V. P. has value when a shocked patient has lost an unknown volume of blood or other body fluids. Intravenous fluids can be administered very rapidly and without risk of overloading the circulation so long as the C. V. P. remains within the normal range. Although a low C. V. P. indicates hypovolaemia, the C. V. P. could be normal if there is hypovolaemia accompanied by vaso-constriction. The technique is useful in the management of abruptio placentae (accidental haemorrhage) when there is often uncertainty over the quantity of blood in the uterus and undertransfusion is a common error. A serious diagnostic error can be avoided by measuring the C. V. P. A patient who is in cardiac failure may have a low arterial blood pressure but will have a high C. V. P. Transfusion could prove fatal to a patient in cardiac failure. C. V. P. monitoring has been used to control the rate of blood transfusion in severely anaemic obstetric patients where the risk of cardiac failure and death from overtransfusion is high. Exchange transfusion has also been used to administer blood safely to severely anaemic obstetric patients.

Intravenous fluids in shock. Restoration of an adequate circulating blood volume by intravenous fluid therapy is the most important aspect of the treatment of shock. The simplest blood substitutes are solutions of water and electrolytes such as normal saline or Ringer's solutions. These solutions will restore the blood volume for a short time only, because within 20 or 30 minutes much of the infused fluid will have passed from the plasma into the extracellular space. Much more effective are plasma and plasma substitutes such as dextran solutions. Dextran is best used in the form of dextran 70 (Macrodex, Lomedex 70) which remains in circulation for up to 48 hours. Dextrans of higher molecular weight were formerly used but were capable of producing a haemorrhagic state and should not be used. Plasma is effective but carries a slight risk of transmitting hepatitis. Haemacel is another effective plasma substitute, most of which remains in the circulation for 3 or 4 hours. Haemacel does not impair coagulation and does not affect cross-matching of blood.

Blood transfusion is traditionally the best treatment for blood loss. The dangers of a mis-matched blood transfusion are worth re-emphasising. The commonest cause of an incompatible blood transfusion is an error in the identification of the bottle or bag of blood or the original specimen sent for grouping and cross-matching. Blood transfusion also carries a risk of transmitting serum hepatitis. There is now a tendency to use a blood substitute for treating haemorrhage of up to 1000 ml and to reserve blood for life-threatening situations.

Blood warming: There is evidence that the rapid transfusion of large volumes of cold blood can cause hypothermia and may cause death from cardiac arrest (ventricular fibrillation). If blood is to be warmed before transfusion then a specially designed blood warmer should be used. This consists of an electrically heated and thermostatically controlled water bath at 38°C. The blood flows through a coil of tubing which is placed in the blood warmer and the blood reaches the patient at a temperature of about 35°C. Attempts to warm blood by placing the bottle or bag in hot water are both inefficient and dangerous because haemolysis may result. Specially designed infra-red blood warmers can warm a whole bottle or bag of blood very rapidly before transfusion. On no account should blood be warmed by any method other than a properly designed blood warmer.

Metabolic acidosis

When an organ or tissue is inadequately supplied with oxygen, either because there is insufficient oxygen in the blood or because the blood flow to the organ is inadequate, the organ does not immediately die from lack of oxygen. Instead the cells remain alive, but with an anaerobic type of metabolism. Normally metabolism is aerobic, oxygen is utilised, metabolism is complete and the end products of metabolism are carbon dioxide and water. Anaerobic metabolism takes place in the absence of oxygen, metabolism is incomplete and the end products are various organic acids such as lactic acid. These acids accumulate in the blood and tissues and when the pH of the blood falls below the normal value of 7.4 a metabolic acidosis exists.

Metabolic acidosis usually develops after any substantial blood loss because the circulation to the various organs and tissues becomes inadequate unless transfusion is immediate and adequate. The patient who is hypotensive, cold and pale is likely to have a metabolic acidosis. The acidosis impairs the function of many organs including the heart and is a predisposition to cardiac arrhythmias and even to cardiac arrest.

A metabolic acidosis is corrected by the administration of sodium bicarbonate solution or T. H. A. M. An 8.4 per cent solution of sodium contains one milliequivalent of sodium bicarbonate per ml of solution. The extent of the acidosis can be measured by the Astrup or other suitable apparatus.

Defibrination and fibrinolysis

Some aspects of this subject are complex and knowledge is incomplete. Fibrinogen is a plasma protein and is the precursor of fibrin, a substance necessary for the formation of normal blood clots. The quantity of fibrinogen in the plasma may be reduced (hypofibrinogenaemia) or the fibrinogen level may fall to zero (afibrinogenaemia) in various obstetric conditions, including abruptio placentae (accidental haemorrhage), amniotic fluid embolism and when a dead fetus has been retained in the uterus for a prolonged period. Defibrination often develops suddenly, the blood fails to clot normally and severe bleeding occurs which is difficult to stop. Defibrination may occur as the result of the excessive utilisation of fibrinogen in the coagulation process. This coagulation consumption process probably occurs in the formation of the large retroplacental haematoma in some cases of abruptio placentae and in the numerous other serious conditions in which disseminated intravascular coagulation may occur. Defibrination may be associated with the presence of excessive amounts of fibrinolysins (substances which break down fibrin). It should be understood that both fibrinolytic and clotting mechanisms exist in the blood and that normally they are in equilibrium, so that intravascular coagulation does not occur. Local clotting can take place at a site of injury where the equilibrium is temporarily upset.

In a condition such as amniotic fluid embolism there is extensive intravascular coagulation in the pulmonary vessels and almost always there is also increased fibrinolytic activity. Increased fibrinolytic activity, although at first sight apparently harmful, may be seen as a potentially beneficial response to intravascular coagulation, tending to limit or even decrease clotting within the lung vessels. It is this clotting process which may kill the patient. Consequently, although anti-fibrinolytic agents such as E. A. C. A. (epsilonaminocaproic acid) and Trasylol are available their use is controversial.

Afibrinogenaemia is likely to cause excessive bleeding from the placental site after delivery or at any surgical procedure. Afibrinogenaemia can be corrected by the injection of fibrinogen or by the infusion of triple strength plasma (prepared by adding 500 ml of water for injection to three units of dried plasma). Here again the decision to correct the haematological abnormality is not straightforward because of the risk of aggravating intravascular coagulation in other organs in certain circumstances. The current tendency is to administer blood to replace that which has been lost and to avoid giving fibrinogen. Heparin may be given to limit intravascular coagulation. It should be realised that haemorrhage at delivery in cases of abruptio placentae is more often due to uterine atony than to a deficiency of fibrinogen and that a fibrinogen deficiency does not always cause bleeding.

Amniotic fluid embolism

Amniotic fluid embolism occurs when liquor amnii enters the mother's veins and lodges as emboli in the blood vessels of the lungs. This serious complication may cause sudden death or acute collapse. Amniotic fluid embolism may occur during Caesarean section, at rupture of the membranes (especially if there is hydramnios) and may occur during labour and delivery, particularly when contractions are violent or there is injury to the uterus or the cervix.

The presence of amniotic fluid and its associated debris in the lungs causes breathlessness, cyanosis, hypotension and tachycardia. Pulmonary oedema develops. The basic lesion in this dramatic complication is widespread coagulation within the pulmonary vessels. The flow of blood through the lungs may be so reduced that death from hypoxia follows. Death may also be caused by pulmonary hypertension and cardiac failure.

Defibrination usually occurs if the patient survives and is probably present in every severe case of amniotic fluid embolism. Excessive fibrinolytic activity often also develops. Uterine haemorrhage is likely and may be torrential and continuous.

A diagnosis of amniotic fluid embolism should be considered in every patient who collapses suddenly during amniotomy, labour, delivery or immediately after delivery.

Treatment depends on the particular features of the individual case. Cyanosis and respiratory distress call for the administration of oxygen. The anaesthetist may improve oxygenation and reduce pulmonary oedema by intermittent positive pressure ventilation and tracheal suction. Haemorrhage will require blood transfusion. The decision to correct a fibrinogen deficiency and excessive fibrinolytic acticity requires good judgement in weighing the risk of increasing the extent of coagulation in the pulmonary blood vessels against the risks of uterine haemorrhage. Heparin may be used to minimise the extent of intravascular coagulation. The present trend is to avoid the administration of fibrinogen and antifibrinolytic agents and to rely on blood transfusions.

Other causes of sudden, severe respiratory distress and shock in the labouring or recently delivered woman are Mendelson's syndrome (after general anaesthesia), pulmonary embolism (clot or air), sickle cell crisis (infarctive crisis) and pulmonary oedema precipitated by intravenous ergometrine in patients with hypertension or mitral stenosis.

Phlebolisis is a very delicate procedure requiring the risk of increasing the risk of coagulation. In the pulmonary blood flow, there are risks of uterine haemorrhage. If pain may be used to minimise the extent of the intravenous coagulation. The present used who aired the administration of the hisopian and the Phlebolisis is the, and of why to all not ten-ficious.

Other doses of further, were respectively liberal and shock flow. During the present, because severe it are not advanced syndrome Later several amount the, reduced, and other with as any sickened time, of followed cross, and pulmonary become presented his anxygrous aponying in patients with illegal and postoperative.

Index